PAIN CONTROL

An open learning programme for healthcare workers

Nan Stalker

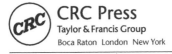

CRC Press
Taylor & Francis Group
Boca Raton London New York

CRC Press is an imprint of the
Taylor & Francis Group, an **informa** business

USING THIS WORKBOOK

The workbook is divided into 'sessions', covering specific subjects.

In the introduction to each learning pack there is a learner profile to help you assess your current knowledge of the subjects covered in each session.

Each session has clear learning objectives. They indicate what you will be able to achieve or learn by completing that session.

Each session has a summary to remind you of the key points of the subjects covered.

Each session contains text, diagrams and learning activities that relate to the stated objectives.

It is important to complete each activity, making your own notes and writing in answers in the space provided. Remember this is your own workbook—you are allowed to write on it.

Now try an example activity.

ACTIVITY

This activity shows you what happens when cells work without oxygen. This really is a physical activity, so please only try it if you are fully fit.

First, raise one arm straight up in the air above your head, and let the other hand rest by your side. Clench both fists tightly, and then open out your fingers wide. Repeat this at the rate of once or twice a second. Try to keep clenching both fists at the same rate. Keep going for about five minutes, and record what you observe.

Stop and rest for a minute. Then try again, with the opposite arm raised this time. Again, record your observations.

[ ]

Suggested timings are given for each activity. These are only a guide. You may like to note how long it took you to complete this activity, as it may help in planning the time needed for working through the sessions.

▼

Time taken on activity   [ ]

▼

Time management is important. While we recognise that people learn at different speeds, this pack is designed to take 15 study hours (your tutor will also advise you). You should allocate time during each week for study.

▼

Take some time now to identify likely periods that you can set aside for study during the week.

	Mon	Tues	Wed	Thurs	Fri	Sat	Sun
am							
pm							
eve							

At the end of the learning pack, there is a learning review to help you assess whether you have achieved the learning objectives.

ACKNOWLEDGEMENTS

Writer: Nan Stalker

Reviewer: Gill Young

Director of programmes: Leslie Mapp

Programmes manager: Caroline Pelletier

Production manager: Stephen Moulds, DSM Partnership

The views expressed are those of the team members and do not necessarily reflect those of The Open Learning Foundation.

The publishers have made all reasonable efforts to contact the holders of copyright material included in this publication.

Radcliffe Medical Press Ltd
18 Marcham Road, Abingdon, Oxon OX14 1AA

British Library Cataloguing in Publication Data

A catalogue record for this book is available from the British Library.

ISBN 1 85775 436 0

Typset by DSM Partnership, London SW18
Printed and bound by TJ International Ltd, Padstow, Cornwall

CONTENTS

INTRODUCTION

This unit focuses primarily on the pharmacological aspects of pain and pain control.

In Session One we revise the topic of neurones. We identify different types of neurone and discuss nerve impulses, neurotransmitters and types of nerve fibre ending.

In Session Two we revise the topic of the structure and function of the brain. We look at the different parts of the brain, and discuss the membranes which cover the brain – the meninges – and the cerebrospinal fluid which protects the brain and the spinal cord.

In Session Three we revise the topic of the structure and function of the spinal cord. We discuss the structure of the spinal cord, and consider peripheral, cranial, spinal and cervical nerves.

In Session Four we revise the topic of voluntary and reflex action and the autonomic nervous system. We start by discussing the function of the central nervous system then discuss voluntary movement and reflex action. We also consider the two parts of the autonomic nervous system: the sympathetic nervous system and the parasympathetic nervous system.

In Session Five we discuss the human experience of pain. We review the history of pain, distinguish between acute and chronic pain, and discuss the modulation of pain.

In Session Six we look at the natural analgesic systems of the human body. We start by discussing the endogenous opioid systems of the body and their role in controlling pain. We then go on to consider how acupuncture draws upon these systems to control pain. We also discuss the issues of referred pain and projected or phantom pain.

In Session Seven we look at the development of chronic pain. We start by looking at how different types of pain are transmitted: in particular, we look at the role played by peripheral sensitisation and hyperalgesia in transmitting chronic pain. We then consider the role of a range of chemical mediators in transmitting pain. Next, we look at drugs that relieve pain by sensitising the nociceptors. Finally, we consider the issue of central sensitisation to pain, and the problem of peripheral nerve damage.

In Session Eight we look at the pharmacology of pain control. We start by defining the most important terms used in the session, then go on to discuss an important group of drugs – the non-steroidal anti-inflammatory drugs or NSAIDs. We consider the mechanisms of NSAIDs, their therapeutic uses and some of the side effects which can be associated with them. Next, we discuss the use of opioids: how they work, their pharmacological properties, their effects, their therapeutic use and the problems of tolerance, withdrawal and dependence. Finally, we consider the use of some other drugs to relieve pain.

In Session Nine we look at the management of pain. We start by considering the World Health Organisation analgesic ladder of pain management, then look in more detail at the use of drugs in pain management, and consider the problems of drug dependence and what is known as 'the pain habit'.

Learning Profile

Below is a list of learning statements for this unit. You can use it as a way of identifying your current knowledge and deciding how the unit can develop your learning. It is for your general guidance only. You will need to check each individual session in more detail to identify specific areas on which you need to focus.

For each of the outcomes listed below, tick the box on the scale which most closely corresponds to your starting point. This will give you a profile of your learning in the areas covered in each session of this unit. The profile is repeated again at the end of this unit as a learning review, and you will be able to check the progress you have made by repeating it again then.

	Not at all	Partly	Quite well	Very well

Session One

I can:

	Not at all	Partly	Quite well	Very well
• describe a typical neurone	❏	❏	❏	❏
• identify different types of neurone and explain their functions	❏	❏	❏	❏
• explain the function of nerve endings	❏	❏	❏	❏
• identify the electrical and chemical factors essential in the functioning of nerve tissue.	❏	❏	❏	❏

Session Two

I can:

	Not at all	Partly	Quite well	Very well
• summarise the functions of the central nervous system	❏	❏	❏	❏
• identify the structure and function of the five main parts of the brain	❏	❏	❏	❏
• explain the function of the ventricles of the brain	❏	❏	❏	❏
• explain the role of the meninges and cerebrospinal fluid.	❏	❏	❏	❏

	Not at all	Partly	Quite well	Very well

Session Three

I can:

- explain the structure and function of the spinal cord

| ❏ | ❏ | ❏ | ❏ |

- identify the peripheral nerves

| ❏ | ❏ | ❏ | ❏ |

- explain the type, function and distribution of the twelve cranial nerves

| ❏ | ❏ | ❏ | ❏ |

- explain the function and route of the spinal nerves.

| ❏ | ❏ | ❏ | ❏ |

Session Four

I can:

- explain the anatomical difference between a voluntary movement and a reflex action

| ❏ | ❏ | ❏ | ❏ |

- explain the roles of the sympathetic and parasympathetic nervous systems

| ❏ | ❏ | ❏ | ❏ |

- identify the functions of the autonomic nervous system.

| ❏ | ❏ | ❏ | ❏ |

Session Five

I can:

- discuss the belief that pain is not a sensation but an emotion

| ❏ | ❏ | ❏ | ❏ |

- identify the different types of pain and their physiological background

| ❏ | ❏ | ❏ | ❏ |

- explain the functions of the two main types of nociceptor

| ❏ | ❏ | ❏ | ❏ |

- discuss the value of superficial electrical stimulus in the control of acute pain

| ❏ | ❏ | ❏ | ❏ |

- evaluate the stimulation of the brain and spinal cord in the control of pain.

| ❏ | ❏ | ❏ | ❏ |

	Not at all	Partly	Quite well	Very well

Session Six

I can:

- describe the endogenous opioid system ❏ ❏ ❏ ❏

- explain the role of the endogenous opioid system in the control of pain ❏ ❏ ❏ ❏

- examine the role of acupuncture in pain control ❏ ❏ ❏ ❏

- explain the pathophysiology of referred pain ❏ ❏ ❏ ❏

- discuss the phenomenon of phantom or projected pain. ❏ ❏ ❏ ❏

Session Seven

I can:

- distinguish between the three categories of pain ❏ ❏ ❏ ❏

- explain the mechanisms which give rise to chronic pain ❏ ❏ ❏ ❏

- discuss the concepts of hyperalgesia and secondary hyperalgesia ❏ ❏ ❏ ❏

- discuss the notion of 'wind-up' as a major feature of chronic pain. ❏ ❏ ❏ ❏

Session Eight

I can:

- identify the three main groups of analgesic drugs ❏ ❏ ❏ ❏

- explain the main functions of non-opioid drugs ❏ ❏ ❏ ❏

- explain the main mechanisms of the opioid drug groups ❏ ❏ ❏ ❏

- discuss the use of adjutant drugs. ❏ ❏ ❏ ❏

	Not at all	Partly	Quite well	Very well

Session Nine

I can:

- describe appropriate drug regimes for the relief of acute and chronic pain ❏ ❏ ❏ ❏

- outline the characteristics of drug dependence in patients being treated with potent analgesics such as morphine ❏ ❏ ❏ ❏

- explain the term 'the pain habit' and discuss how this situation can be prevented ❏ ❏ ❏ ❏

- describe ways in which 'wind-up' can be avoided in surgical and terminal pain. ❏ ❏ ❏ ❏

SESSION ONE

Neurones

Introduction

In this session we revise the topic of neurones. We identify different types of neurone, and discuss nerve impulses, neurotransmitters and types of nerve fibre ending.

Session objectives

When you have completed this session you should be able to:

● describe a typical neurone

● identify different types of neurone and explain their functions

● explain the function of nerve endings

● identify the electrical and chemical factors essential in the functioning of nerve tissue.

1: Nervous tissue

The nervous system is the system of communication between the various parts of the body. It can be compared to a simple telephone system in which the brain is comparable to the central switchboard, the spinal cord is comparable to the main cable and the nerves are comparable to the telephone wires, ending in receivers and dischargers of messages in the body tissue. It is a two-way system with messages being transmitted between the brain and the body tissue via the neural network. Like the skeletal and muscular systems, the nervous system is made up of a special tissue – the nervous tissue.

ACTIVITY 1 // ALLOW 5 MINUTES

Name the two component parts of nervous tissue and identify the name given collectively to the two parts.

Commentary

The two component parts of the nervous tissue are **nerve cells** and **nerve fibres**. Collectively, the cell and its fibres are called a **neurone**.

The neurone is the unit on which the nervous system is built. Cells and fibres are bound together by a special type of connective tissue known as neuroglia – this binds them into a solid but very soft and delicate tissue.

ACTIVITY 2 // ALLOW 5 MINUTES

Each cell has one long fibre and several short fibres. Name the long fibre and the short fibres and in one or two sentences identify their function.

Commentary

The long fibre is called the **axon**, and the short fibre is called the **dendrite**. The axon carries impulses from a cell and at its ending passes the impulses on to another nerve cell or dendrite, or to tissue. The dendrite picks up the impulse or message and carries the impulse or message to a cell.

Nerve cells are grouped together to form grey matter. Grey matter is found at the periphery of the brain, the centre of the spinal cord and in the ganglia. (A ganglion is a small mass of isolated nerve cells.)

Nerve fibres are grouped together to form the white matter of the nervous system. White matter is found at the centre of the brain, the periphery of the spinal cord and in the nerves.

A nerve is simply a bundle of nerve fibres bound together by connective tissue. Whiteness of a nerve fibre is due to its protective sheath, which makes a marked difference in colour of the tissue, readily obvious to the naked eye.

The nerve sheath consists of two coats, an outer coat of connective tissue called neurilemma and a thick inner fatty sheath called the myelin sheath. This fatty sheath is interrupted at intervals and the outer neurilemma dips in and forms notches called Nodes of Ranvier.

ACTIVITY 3 // ALLOW 5 MINUTES

Identify and explain the three main functions of the myelin sheath.

Commentary

The three main functions of the myelin sheath are as follows.

- **Protection** from pressure and injury.

- **Nutrition**. As the fibres may be of great length, varying from 2.5 cm to 7.5 cm or more, the distal part of the fibre may be a long way from the cell which controls the nutrition of its protoplasm. For example, nerve cells in the lumbar region of the spinal cord give off nerve fibres to the foot and may be more than a metre in length. The sheath may help to nourish the fibre.

- **Insulation**. It is also suggested that the sheath acts like the casing of an electric wire, so that impulses carried by the nerve are not transmitted to adjacent nerves or tissues except through the end of a fibre.

The nerve cell and its fibres are one living unit, and if the fibre is cut off from the cell it will die, as it is the cell which contains the nucleus and the protoplasms of the fibre. Conversely, if the cell and the portion of the fibre attached to it remain alive, a new fibre can grow from the severed end provided the neurilemma remains intact.

It should be remembered that the fibre will not grow through fibrous scar tissue of a wound; it will, however, grow along an old nerve sheath. As a result, the nerve supply can be restored if a nerve is cut, though it will take time for the nerve fibre to grow, as these fibres, though often short, can be as much as a metre in length. It will, however, take much longer for the newly grown fibre to learn to function fully. If the nerve cell is destroyed by injury or disease the fibre will also die. If this happens, neither the cell nor the fibre can be replaced.

ACTIVITY 4 // ALLOW 5 MINUTES

Draw and label a diagram of a neurone.

Commentary

Your diagram should be similar to that shown in Figure 1, below.

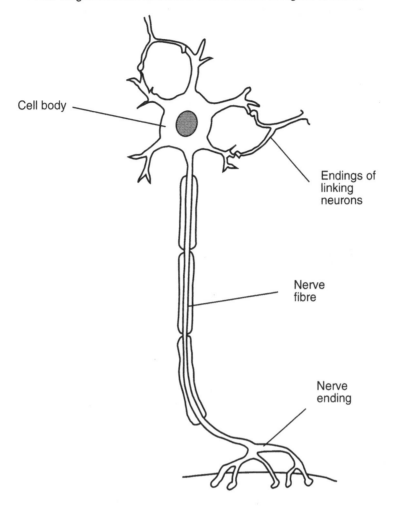

Cell body

Endings of
linking
neurons

Nerve
fibre

Nerve
ending

Figure 1: Diagram of neurone

2: Types of neurone

ACTIVITY 5   // ALLOW 5 MINUTES

Identify the two main types of neurone and their functions, and give examples of
these functions.

Commentary

Efferent neurones carry impulses from the brain to the tissues. Examples include motor neurones, which supply the muscles and produce movement, and secretory neurones, which supply the glands and produce secretions. Figure 2, below, shows an efferent neurone.

Afferent neurones carry impulses to the brain from the tissues. These give rise to sensations such as touch, pain, heat or cold, and are sometimes known as sensory neurones. Figure 3, below, shows an afferent neurone.

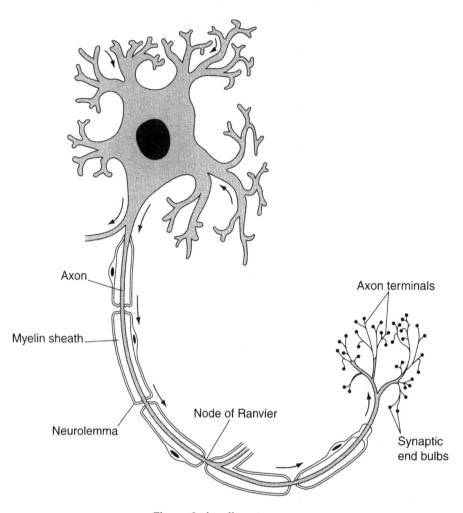

Figure 2: An efferent neurone

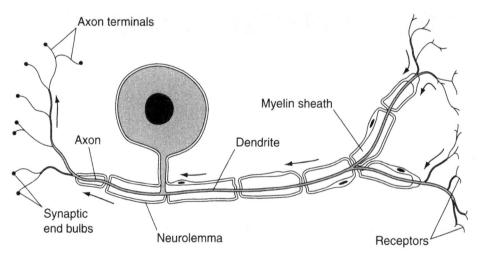

Figure 3: An afferent (sensory) neurone

If there is loss of nerve supply to tissues then necrosis of the tissue occurs; healing cannot take place unless the nerve supply is restored. There are also associate or connective neurones which run between the efferent and afferent neurones in the brain and the spinal cord. These connector neurones, to relate them to our telephone system, are like internal telephones in a building such as a hospital.

The neurone shown in Figure 1, earlier, is a typical neurone, consisting of a cell giving off many dendrites and one axon. Sensory neurones have a different structure: they have specialised nerve endings in the skin by which sensations are picked up. Fibres run from these nerve endings into the vertebral column and they are protected by the bone. The delicate cell is joined to the fibre by T-like connections; from this cell the fibre runs on into the cord to pass the impulse to the afferent and associate nerve cells of the cord. These neurones are called unipolar neurones.

ACTIVITY 6   ALLOW 5 MINUTES

Discuss the method of communication between the axon of one neurone with the dendrites of another nerve cell.

Commentary

The axon normally ends in a tree-like branching by which the stimuli carried by the axon are passed on to the dendrites of another nerve cell. The fibre ends in nervous tissue and passes the impulse on to another nerve cell, the axon of which must communicate with the dendrites of another nerve cell for the passage of the impulse to take place; this point is called the synapse.

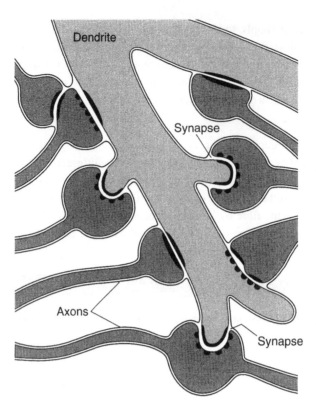

Figure 4: A synapse

A synapse permits passage of an impulse in one direction only and offers some resistance to its passage. However, in the pharmacology of pain it must be remembered that the dendrites of the adjacent neurones do not actually touch the axon. The impulse passes across the synapse because of a chemical substance, acetylcholine. This substance is released at the junction, which then stimulates the dendrites of another neurone or neurones.

3: The nerve impulse

One of the ways in which substances may enter and exit a cell is via the process of osmosis. In order for this process to occur the cell membrane has to be semi-permeable. This means that cell walls have a variety of 'gates' through which various substances are allowed to pass. There are many types of gate, each one allowing a particular substance through.

On the outside surface of a membrane there are receptor zones which influence the gates in a variety of ways. They may open the gate, allowing substances to pass through, or they may alter the structure of the gate and influence the internal structure of the membrane.

When a nerve cell is stimulated at any point, its membrane is affected and some of the gates open, allowing sodium and potassium ions to move in and out. Before the gates open, the distribution of these ions, which carry an electrical charge, produces a specific charge across the membrane. When the gate opens the charge changes. This affects the adjacent section of membrane and causes gates to open there too, and so on across the nerve cell and down to the nerve end. This is the nerve impulse – a self-generating wave of electrical activity passing from the point of stimulation to the nerve ending.

4: Neurotransmitters

The nerve impulse is a form of electrical activity. The gap between the nerve end and the next cell is a fluid-filled space – the synapse. The impulse cannot jump across the gap like a spark in an electrical circuit. It has to be converted into chemical activity in order to cross that space. This is where neurotransmitters come in. These chemicals are released when the electrical impulse reaches one side of a synapse. They pass across it and influence the membrane on the other side, causing changes in that membrane leading to the initiation of electrical activity there. So the impulse travels from one cell to the next.

A similar process occurs when the nerve ending synapses with a structure such as an endocrine gland, over which it has control. So, throughout the nervous system and the structures it controls we have the same pattern recurring: electrical activity alternating with chemical activity. This process begins when a sensory nerve ending receives a stimulus.

For a more detailed account of how a synapse functions you should read *Resource 1* from the *Resources Section* which has been downloadad from the following web site http://faculty.washington.edu/chudler/synapse.html. You might like to explore this web site yourself.

5: Types of nerve fibre ending

ACTIVITY 7   **// ALLOW 5 MINUTES**

Name and describe the functions of the two main types of nerve fibre ending.

Commentary

The two main types of nerve fibre ending are:

- motor nerve endings
- sensory nerve endings.

Motor nerve endings give off stimuli to the muscles producing contractions – these are called motor end plates. Each muscle fibre is stimulated through a single motor end plate.

Sensory nerve endings pick up impulses and carry them into the spinal cord and brain. These are the afferent or sensory neurones, which give rise to sensations, but it must be remembered that many of these sensations remain below the level of consciousness.

These nerve endings in the tissues are often peculiar in structure. Some of them are simple tree-like branchings similar to the fibre endings found in nerve tissue. On the other hand, motor nerve endings branch but the tip of each branch carries a disc-shaped plate in the actual muscle fibre. This is the motor end plate.

Nerves of touch in the skin end in little round bodies which when sectioned look like an onion under a microscope – touch and tactile corpuscles which are stimulated on pressure. Nerve endings of sight end in cone or rod-shaped cells in the retina of the eye, and these are stimulated by light. The nerves of hearing end in hair-bearing cells in the ear which are affected by sound. Nerves of taste end in taste buds in the tongue.

The nature of the impulses carried by nerve tissue is electrical. However, as in an electric battery chemical reactions are associated with the passing of an electric current, so in the body chemical changes associated with potassium and chloride ions accompany the electrical impulse. It is important to remember that the function of nerve tissue has both an electrical and a chemical factor – in the pharmacology of pain it is often a chemical imbalance which influences pain, as we have seen above.

Reading *Resource 2* will help you to revise how neurones transmit messages through electrochemical processes.

Before you move on to Session Two, check that you have achieved the objectives given at the beginning of this session and, if not, review the appropriate sections.

The brain

Introduction

In this session we revise the topic of the structure and function of the brain, look at the different parts of the brain, and discuss the membranes which cover the brain – the meninges – and the cerebrospinal fluid which protects the brain and the spinal cord.

Session objectives

When you have completed this session you should be able to:

● summarise the functions of the central nervous system

● identify the structure and function of the five main parts of the brain

● explain the function of the ventricles of the brain

● explain the role of the meninges and cerebrospinal fluid.

1: The central nervous system

ACTIVITY 1 // **ALLOW 5 MINUTES**

Summarise the functions of the central nervous system.

Commentary

The central nervous system contracts the voluntary muscles of the head, trunk and limbs and is responsible for all movement in them and for all sensation in skin, muscle, bones and joints and the special sense organs.

The central nervous system supplies nerves to the limbs and to the structures which form the walls of the cavities of the head and trunk and the covering muscles and skin.

Nerves given off by the brain and spinal cord, which go to the outer part of the body are called peripheral nerves to distinguish them from the nerves supplying the internal organs.

The central nervous system is present at a very early stage when the developing fertilised ovum consists of a mass of cells arranged in an outer, middle and inner layer, with a groove appearing on the surface – this groove is known as the neural groove. The outer layer of cells in which it is formed develops into the skin, while the middle layer forms muscles, bone and other connective tissues, and the inner layer forms the lining membranes of hollow internal organs.

ACTIVITY 2   // ALLOW 5 MINUTES

Briefly outline the physiological development of the neural groove.

Commentary

The neural groove gradually turns into a canal, its walls growing up and joining round it. The walls of the canal develop to form the cord which always has a lining canal running through the centre of it. At the upper end, where the head is to develop, the canal becomes enlarged and the walls of the enlarged cavity develop to form the brain. Although the groove forms on the surface of the embryo, the other layers gradually grow up around it, so that the brain and spinal cord become very well protected from injury before birth.

Figure 5 shows how the various elements of the central nervous system and the peripheral nervous system relate to one another.

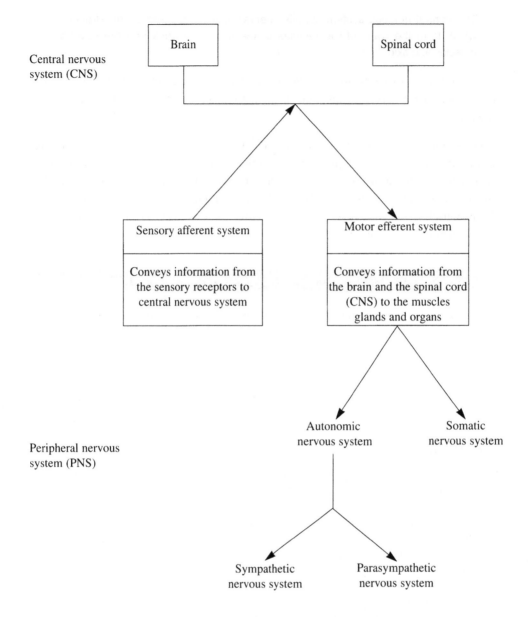

Figure 5: The nervous system

2: The brain

When fully developed the brain is a large organ filling the cranial cavity, and can weigh anything between one and four kilograms. Its large size compared to the total body weight is one of the main anatomical differences between humans and other animals.

The brain is a complex organ. Early in its development its cavity becomes divided by constrictures into three parts – forebrain, midbrain and hindbrain. From the walls of these three parts the fully developed brain is formed, the cavities persisting and being called ventricles.

ACTIVITY 3   **//**   **ALLOW 5 MINUTES**

Name the five main parts of the brain.

Commentary

The five main parts of the brain are:

- cerebrum
- cerebellum
- midbrain
- medulla oblongata.
- pons Varolii

Figure 6 shows the location of the main parts of the brain.

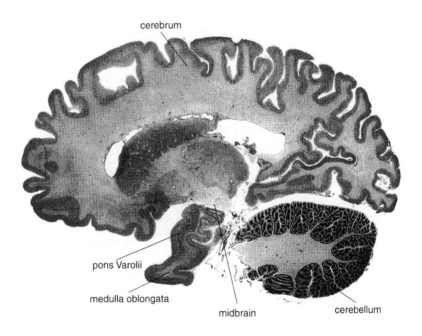

Figure 6: The main parts of the brain

The cerebrum

The cerebrum fills the vault of the cranium from the level of the eyebrows in front to the occiput at the back. It is divided into two hemispheres – right and left – by a deep central fissure, the longitudinal cerebral fissure. These hemispheres control the opposite sides of the body, so that disease of the right side of the cerebrum affects the left side of the body and disease of the left side of the cerebrum affects the right side of the body. Each hemisphere contains a small cavity or ventricle, known as the right and left lateral ventricles.

Each hemisphere is subdivided into lobes which correspond approximately with the bones of the cranium. The chief lobes are:

● the frontal lobe

● the parietal lobe

● the occipital lobe

● the temporal lobe.

Figure 7 shows the location of the most important lobes.

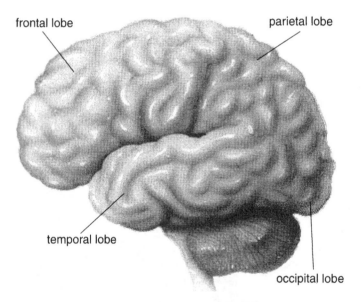

Figure 7: The main lobes of the brain

These lobes are divided from one another by deep fissures known as sulci. The central sulcus divides the frontal and parietal lobes; the lateral sulcus divides the temporal lobe from the frontal and parietal lobes; and the perieto-occipital sulcus passes downwards and forwards from the back of the hemispheres.

The cerebrum consists of grey matter or nerve cells on the surface, and white matter or nerve fibres in the centre. The surface is convoluted: this means that it is thrown into ridges and depressions. This greatly increases its mass and therefore increases the amount of grey matter, or nerve cells, which are the foundation of our mental capacities. Convolutions are more extensive than in the lower order animals. This further increases the possibilities of mental development. The grey matter on the surface of the cortex of the cerebrum contains many important nerve centres.

ACTIVITY 4 // **ALLOW 10 MINUTES**

Identify and discuss the functions of the cerebral cortex.

Commentary

The cerebrum contains many important nerve centres, which make it not only the largest but also the most highly developed part of the brain. These centres include the following:

- **motor centres** control all the voluntary muscles of the muscular system

- **sensory centres** interpret sensory impulses, which give sensation to the skin and to a lesser extent to the muscles, bones and joints

- **centres of special sense**: sight, hearing, smell, taste and touch

- **centres of higher mental powers**: consciousness, memory, intelligence and reasoning power.

The position of these centres within the lobes are, to a large extent, known. Motor centres lie in the frontal lobe in the front of the central sulcus. Those for the lower limbs are at the top, next come those of the trunk, upper limbs, neck and head, extending outwards and downwards in front of the fissure. The motor centres for the eye lie further forward. (For this reason, frontal headache may be due to eye problems.) The speech centre also lies in the frontal lobe, normally in the left cerebral hemisphere.

Sensory centres for the limbs, trunk and head lie in the parietal lobe just behind the central sulcus in positions corresponding to the motor areas. The centre of sight is in the occipital lobe, and the centres of smell and hearing are in the temporal lobe.

Types of fibre

White matter consists of nerve fibres running to, from and between the cells of the cortex.

Motor fibres run from the motor centres of the cortex out through the base of the brain into the spinal cord, carrying impulses from the brain.

Sensory fibres run in from the base of the brain to the sensory centres of the cortex. These carry impulses to the cerebral nerve centres.

Association or connector fibres run from one nerve centre to another and from hemisphere to hemisphere linking them to one another, so that the various centres of the brain can work as a whole and communicate with one another. A mass of connector neurones made up of fibres linking the two hemispheres form a bridge-like structure at the base of the fissure which separates the hemispheres from one another: this is called the corpus callosum.

Returning to our telephone exchange analogy from Session One, the nerve endings not only receive messages, they also store them so that they can be recalled, giving rise to memory, and can be used as a guide to the action to be taken when a similar stimulus is received again.

Nerve fibres run towards a point at the centre of the base of the cerebrum, where they form stalks which pass to the midbrain. Between them in the base of the cerebrum is a small cavity – the third ventricle – into which the lateral ventricles lead. There is also a small amount of grey matter, which consists almost entirely of sensory cells. These cells receive the stimuli which are being brought into the brain by the afferent nerve fibres, and relay the stimuli on via fresh neurones to the nerve centres of the cortex. This grey matter is sometimes referred to as cerebral or basal nuclei.

The cerebral nuclei include the thalami on either side, forming the lateral walls of the third ventricle. These are mainly made up of sensory cells relaying sensory stimuli to the cortex.

The corpus striatum lies laterally to the thalamus on either side. It is separated from it by the internal capsule which consists of the conveying tracts of motor and sensory nerve fibres between the thalamus and corpus striatum, running to and from the cerebral cortex. The corpus striatum is largely a motor relay station and is so called because nerve fibres pass through it, giving it a striped appearance.

The pyramidal tract and many other motor and sensory tracts run in the narrow internal capsule. This is the area usually involved when the patient has a cerebral vascular accident. The hypothalamus exercises influence over the autonomic nervous system. It contains the heat-regulating centre and communicates with the posterior lobe of the pituitary gland.

The midbrain

The midbrain consists of two thick stalk-like bands of thick matter which pass out from the base of the cerebrum and run into the pons Varolii. It contains some grey matter and a fine canal, called the aqueduct of the midbrain, runs through it from the third ventricle to the fourth ventricle, which lies behind the cerebellum, behind the pons Varolii with the medulla oblongata in front. The white matter consists of motor and sensory fibres running from and to the nerve centres of the cerebral cortex and cerebral nuclei.

The cerebellum

The cerebellum is smaller than the cerebrum and lies below it and towards the back.

ACTIVITY 5 // ALLOW 5 MINUTES

Describe the structure of the cerebellum and discuss its function.

Commentary

The cerebellum is sometimes known as the hindbrain, and is similar in structure to the cerebrum. There are three pairs of cerebellar stalks or peduncles joining it to the midbrain above, the pons Varolii in front and the medulla oblongata below. Impulses passing into the cerebellum via these peduncles keep it informed of the state of the muscles. Its functions are not completely understood. However, it is known to be responsible for maintaining equilibrium, muscle coordination and muscle tone. Destruction of the cerebellum by disease results in loss of power to coordinate muscular actions, with the result that the patient cannot stand or walk steadily, but staggers.

The pons Varolii

The pons Varolii consists almost entirely of white matter and forms the link joining the various parts of the brain to one another.

ACTIVITY 6 **// ALLOW 5 MINUTES**

Describe the two main parts of the pons Varolii.

Commentary

The pons Varolii consists of:

- a bridge-like portion, joining one hemisphere of the cerebellum to the other – this is the middle cerebellar peduncle

- a mass of fibres running from the cerebrum and midbrain above, flowing under the bridge-like structure.

Two thick stalk-like bands of white matter pass out from the base of the cerebrum. They consist of motor and sensory fibres running from and to the nerve centres of the cortex. These bands of white matter are the continuation of the nerve fibres which pass through the midbrain and the pons, filling in the gap under the bridge-like portion completely, and run on into the medulla oblongata or cerebellum below. The pons Varolii therefore joins the cerebrum above through the midbrain to the medulla oblongata and cerebellum below, and also joins the two hemispheres of the cerebellum to one another.

The medulla oblongata

The medulla oblongata joins the pons Varolii above to the spinal cord below. The link between the brain and the spinal cord is sometimes referred to as the spinal bulb. This is of similar structure to the spinal cord but slightly thicker. It lies within the foramen magnum at the base of the brain.

Most of the motor fibres cross here, so that the left side of the brain controls the right side of the body and the right side of the brain controls the left side of the body.

Vital centres

These are respiratory, cardiac and vaso-motor centres which are essential to the continuance of life. Conscious life is dependent on the higher centres of the cerebrum. These may be thrown temporarily out of action during sleep and unconsciousness, but the lower centres of the medulla oblongata must continue to function or death ensues at once. Injury here causes instant death.

Reflex centres

These centres in the medulla oblongata control food and air passages and produce automatic reflex actions such as swallowing, vomiting, coughing and sneezing.

ACTIVITY 7 // ALLOW 5 MINUTES

The brain contains four cavities known as ventricles. The first and second ventricles are the lateral ventricles. Identify the location of the third and fourth ventricles.

Commentary

The third ventricle lies in the midline of the base of the cerebrum. The fourth ventricle lies between the pons, the medulla oblongata and the cerebellum. These ventricles communicate with one another and with the subarachnoid space, and contain cerebrospinal fluid.

3: The meninges and cerebrospinal fluid

The meninges

The brain and spinal cord are covered by three membranes known as the meninges.

ACTIVITY 8 // ALLOW 5 MINUTES

Identify and discuss the functions of the three membranes which are known as the meninges.

Commentary

Dura mater: this outer layer is a tough fibrous membrane, itself composed of two layers. The outer layer is attached to the inner surface of the skull, forming the periostium. However, the two layers are separate where they enclose a venous sinus. At the foramen magnum the outer layer continues as periostium on the outer surface of the skull and only the inner layer passes down the spinal cord. One portion – the tentorium cerebelli – dips in between the cerebrum and cerebellum. Another portion – the falx cerebri – dips down between the two hemispheres of the cerebrum. The dura mater helps to support and protect the delicate brain substance.

Arachnoid mater: this is a delicate serous membrane lying close beneath the dura mater and dipping down with it between the main portions of the brain. The arachnoid forms a tube within the dura mater. Between the arachnoid mater and the pia mater is the sub-arachnoid space.

Pia mater: this is a delicate membrane, richly supplied with blood vessels, which covers the actual surface of the brain and dips down into all its convolutions. It carries the blood supply to the underlying brain.

Cerebrospinal fluid

This is a clear watery fluid which collects between the arachnoid mater and the pia mater in the sub-arachnoid space, into which it oozes from the choroid plexus in the lateral ventricles of the brain.

It protects the brain and spinal cord, acting as a watery barrier between the delicate nerve tissue and the lining walls of the cavities in which the structures lie. It also nourishes and cleanses, washing away waste and toxic substances. The fluid is absorbed by the arachnoid granulations in the venous sinus. The brain is therefore protected by the hair, tough scalp, cranial bones, dura mater and cerebrospinal fluid.

Before you move on to Session Three, check that you have achieved the objectives given at the beginning of this session and, if not, review the appropriate sections.

SESSION THREE

The spinal cord

Introduction

In this session we revise the topic of the structure and function of the spinal cord. We discuss the structure of the spinal cord and consider peripheral, cranial, spinal and cervical nerves.

Session objectives

When you have completed this session you should be able to:

● explain the structure and function of the spinal cord

● identify the peripheral nerves

● explain the type, function and distribution of the twelve cranial nerves

● explain the function and route of the spinal nerves.

1: The structure of the spinal cord

This is a cylinder of nerve tissue, about the thickness of the little finger and from 38 to 45 centimetres long. It joins the medulla oblongata above and runs down the spinal canal to the level of the base of the body of the first lumbar vertebra, where it ends in a bunch of nerves called the cauda equina. These nerves pass out from the lumbar and sacral regions of the vertebral column.

The spinal cord varies somewhat in thickness, swelling out in both the cervical and lumbar regions, when it gives off the large nerve supply to the limbs. These are called the cervical and lumbar enlargements. The cord has a deep cleft both back and front, so that it is almost completely divided into right and left sides like the cerebrum.

The white matter is found on the outside or surface of the cord, and is made up of nerve fibres running between the cord and the brain. You should note that these fibres do not run to the body tissues.

White matter contains:

- motor or efferent fibres running down from the motor centre of the cerebrum and the cerebellum to the motor cells of the cord

- sensory or afferent fibres running up the cord from the sensory cells of the cord to the sensory centres of the brain.

The grey matter is found inside the spinal cord and forms an 'H' shape. The portions which project forwards are called the anterior horns and the portions projecting backwards are called the posterior horns.

The anterior horns consist of motor cells which give off motor fibres to the muscles of the trunk and limbs. These fibres run out and from the motor fibres of the spinal nerves. A motor impulse from the motor centre in the brain is carried by an efferent fibre down to the motor cell in the spinal cord. The motor cells in the brain and the fibres which run from them to the anterior horns of the cord are called upper motor neurones. The motor cells in the cord and the fibres which run from them to the muscles are called lower motor neurones.

The posterior horns consist of sensory cells. These give off sensory fibres which run up the cord to the centres at the base of the brain; these pass on the impulses they receive to the sensory centres of the cerebrum. Sensory fibres from body tissues run into and end in the posterior horns of the cord, bringing in impulses from the tissue to the sensory cells and to the connective cells of the posterior horns.

Impulses are brought in by afferent fibres from the tissues to the cells of the cord, which pick up the impulses and pass them up the cord to the sensory centres of the brain, producing sensation. Sensation of pain and temperature cross at once to the opposite side of the cord; other sensations cross at higher levels.

ACTIVITY 1 // ALLOW 5 MINUTES

Identify the two main functions of the spinal cord.

Commentary

The spinal cord:

- is the link between the brain and the nerves supplying the outer part of the trunk and the limbs

- is an important centre of reflex action.

2: Nerves

The peripheral nerves

Nerves extend from the brain and the spinal cord. There are:

● twelve pairs of cranial nerves

● thrity-one pairs of spinal nerves arising from the cord.

The cranial nerves

These supply the organs of the head and neck. They are as a rule, either motor or sensory, but some are mixed. They include the nerves of smell, taste, sight and hearing, and the vagus nerve. The vagus nerve supplies organs in the neck, thorax and abdomen; its branches wander about the trunk. It assists in the formation of the autonomic nervous system.

ACTIVITY 2	**// ALLOW 30 MINUTES**

Identify the twelve cranial nerves by name, by type, and by function and distribution.

Commentary

Name	Type	Function and distribution
Olfactory	Sensory	Supplies the nose and is the nerve of smell.
Optic	Sensory	Supplies the eye and is the nerve of sight.
Oculomotor	Motor	Supplies the muscles moving the eye and within the eye.
Trochlear	Motor	Supplies the superior oblique muscle of the eye.
Trigeminal	Motor and sensory	Supplies muscles of mastication with three sensory branches to the orbits, upper and lower jaws: ophthalmic, maxillary and mandibular.
Abducen	Motor	Supplies only the lateral rectus muscle of the eye.
Facial	Motor and sensory	Supplies muscles of facial expression and supplies taste to the anterior part of the tongue.
Auditory	Sensory	Supplies the ear and is the nerve of hearing and balance.
Glosso-pharyngeal	Mixed	Supplies the posterior part of the tongue and pharynx and is the nerve of taste. Supplies motor fibres to the pharynx.
Vagus	Mixed	Supplies internal organs, controlling secretion and movement. Also supplies the larynx.
Accessory	Motor	Supplies the muscles of the neck. Also supplies most of the muscles of the pharynx and the soft palate and one branch joins the vagus to supply the pharynx.
Hypoglossal	Motor	Supplies the muscles of the tongue.

It may help you to think of pain which either you or a patient has encountered. An example would be earache. This relates to the auditory nerve; people often have a problem with balance when they have earache.

The facial nerve is the nerve affected in facial paralysis. It leaves the cranium with the vertibulo-cochlear nerve and runs through the ear, so it may become infected or injured in diseases of and operations in the ear. An example of this is Bell's palsy.

When the vagus and accessory nerves are affected by injury or disease the muscles involved in swallowing are paralysed. There is danger of asphyxia, as neither natural secretions nor food and drink can be swallowed and are liable to be inhaled into the air passage. This occurs in the bulbar form of poliomyelitis. It may also cause complete blockage of the airway or aspiration pneumonia.

The spinal nerves

The spinal nerves supply the muscles of the trunk and limbs with the power of movement, and give sensation to the skin and to a lesser extent the muscles, bones and joints around the spine.

There are thrity-one pairs of spinal nerves, which are mixed nerves: this means that they contain both motor and sensory fibres. They arise from the spinal cord by two roots:

● anterior or motor roots

● posterior or sensory roots.

Anterior or motor roots consist of fibre coming from motor cells of the anterior horns. Posterior or sensory roots consist of sensory fibres bringing in sensory stimuli from the skin and, to a lesser extent, from other tissue. The fibres run into the vetrectial canal and from the posterior roots of spinal nerves. On each root is a ganglion which is visible as a marked swelling and which is called the posterior root ganglion. This consists of the cells of these fibres which have the protection of the spinal column and which are joined by a T-shaped branch to the fibre. From the ganglion the fibre runs on and enters the posterior horn of the spinal cord, where it ends in a widely spread tree-like branching. This branching passes on the stimuli brought in by the fibre to the sensory cells of the cord on the same or opposite side.

ACTIVITY 3   **// ALLOW 10 MINUTES**

Identify the cervical, thoracic, lumbar, sacral and coccygeal nerves by distribution.

Commentary

There are eight pairs of cervical nerves, one above the atlas and one below each of the cervical vertebrae.

There are twelve pairs of thoracic nerves, one below each of the thoracic vertebrae.

There are five pairs of lumbar nerves, five pairs of sacral nerves and one pair of coccygeal nerves. These are derived from the cauda equina.

The spinal nerves give off short posterior branches which supply the muscles of the back of the neck and trunk, and long anterior branches which provide the nerves of the limbs and the sides and front of the trunk.

In some regions these nerves branch as soon as they leave the spinal canal, with the branches joining up to form nerves supplying the various muscles. This inter-branching is called a plexus. Plexus are found in all regions except the thoracic region.

Cervical nerves

Cervical nerves come from two plexus:

- the cervical plexus, supplying the muscles of the neck and shoulder and giving off the phrenic nerve supplying the diaphragm.

- the brachial plexus, supplying the upper limbs. This plexus gives off three main nerves.

ACTIVITY 4   **// ALLOW 5 MINUTES**

Identify the route and function of the three main nerves of the brachial plexus.

Commentary

The three main nerves of the brachial plexus are as follows.

- The **radial nerve**. This runs round the back of the humerus and down the outside of the forearm. It supplies the extensor muscles of the elbow, wrist and hand.

- The **ulnar** and **median nerves**. These run down the inside and middle of the limbs respectively and supply the flexor muscles of the wrist and hand. The ulnar nerve crosses in the groove between the back surface of the internal epicondyle of the humerus and the olecranon process.

- The **thoracic nerves**. These supply the muscles of the chest and the main part of the abdominal wall.

The lumbar nerves form the lumbar plexus. This branches off into one main nerve, the femoral nerve. This runs down beside the psoas muscle under the inguinal ligament into the front of the thigh, supplying the muscle in this region. The lumbar plexus also branches off to the lower abdominal wall.

The sacral nerves, with branches from the fourth and fifth lumbar nerves, form the sacral plexus, which gives rise to one large nerve: the sciatic nerve. It is the longest nerve in the body. It leaves the pelvis via the sciatic notch, runs across the back of the hip joint and down the back of the thigh, supplying the muscles there. It divides above the knee into two main branches. These are:

- the popliteal nerve, which supplies the muscles of the front of the leg and the foot

- the tibial nerve, which supplies the muscles of the back of the leg.

The sciatic nerve therefore supplies the whole of the leg below the knee except for a small sensory branch from the femoral nerve.

ACTIVITY 5 // ALLOW 5 MINUTES

What is a common cause of back pain? Where does the patient often complain the pain is?

Commentary

A common cause of back pain is **sciatica**. Sciatica is a type of neuritis characterised by pain along the path of the sciatic nerve or its branches. Because of its length and size, the sciatic nerve is vulnerable to many types of injury. As a result of inflammation or injury the patient often complains of pain which may travel from the back or thigh down its length into the leg, foot and toes.

The coccygeal nerves, together with branches from the lower sacral nerves, form a second small plexus on the back of the pelvic cavity. This plexus supplies the muscles and skin in that area. Examples include muscles of the perineal body, the internal sphincter of the anus, the skin and other tissues of the external genitals and the perineum.

Both the sacral and coccygeal nerves also have branches to the sympathetic ganglia in the pelvic area.

Before you move on to Session Four, check that you have achieved the objectives given at the beginning of this session and, if not, review the appropriate sections.

Voluntary and reflex action and the autonomic nervous system

Introduction

In this session we revise the topic of voluntary and reflex action and the autonomic nervous system. We start by discussing the function of the central nervous system and then discuss voluntary movement and reflex action. We also consider the two parts of the autonomic nervous system: the sympathetic nervous system and the parasympathetic nervous system.

Session objectives

When you have completed this session you should be able to:

- explain the anatomical difference between a voluntary movement and a reflex action

- explain the roles of the sympathetic and parasympathetic nervous systems

- identify the functions of the autonomic nervous system.

1: The function of the central nervous system

Identify five specific functions of the central nervous system.

Commentary

The central nervous system:

- is the seat of all sensation

- controls all movement of voluntary muscle

- is the seat of all special senses

- is the seat of higher mental powers – reasoning and so on

- controls vital functions of respiration and circulation, the controlling centres being located in the hypothalamus and the medulla oblongata.

2: Voluntary movement

Voluntary movement occurs as a result of stimuli produced at will in the motor centres of the brain. The stimuli are transmitted by motor fibres, via the cord and nerves, to the muscles to produce contractions.

Reflexes are fast responses to the internal or external changes in the environment, allowing the body to maintain homeostasis. Reflexes are associated with both skeletal muscle contraction and with those of the body systems such as heart rate, respiration and urination. A spinal reflex occurs when the action is carried out by the spinal cord, whilst reflexes that result in skeletal muscle movement are known as somatic reflexes. An autonomic reflex action is one which causes involuntary muscle to contract: for example, cardiac muscle and smooth muscle.

The spinal column and the brain are constantly receiving sensory information from body tissue. However, we only become conscious of a sensation if it is passed along to be interpreted by a sensory centre. When the stimuli reach the sensory centres of the cerebrum they then produce sensations of which we are conscious. Should the stimulus continue to synapse with and stimulate a motor cell a reflex action is produced.

3: Reflex action

Reflex action occurs as a result of the stimulation of the motor cells by stimuli transmitted by afferent neurones from the tissues. Incoming stimuli can therefore, in addition to causing sensation, give rise to action. They only produce sensation if they are passed on to the sensory centres of the brain. On the other hand, in the cord and in the brain they may stimulate the motor cells and give rise to action – reflex action. Sensory stimuli are passed into the cord and brain from the tissues all the time. If these stimuli reach the sensory centres of the cortex of the cerebrum and stimulate them, they produce sensations of which we are conscious. If they stimulate motor cells they produce reflex action. For example, touching something hot causes immediate withdrawal of the body part.

The sensory stimulus is carried into the spinal cord by sensory fibres. It is transmitted to connector fibres to the motor cells of the anterior horn, and exits via the motor fibres to the muscles. In the case of knee jerk, the sensory stimulus is transported into the lumbar region of the spinal cord by afferent fibres and stimulates the motor cells which control the quadriceps.

The reason for the reflex being more marked when the cord is cut off from the brain is that central centres have an inhibiting effect on reflex action. Reflex action is not produced by the will; it is a response to environment and is the only type of action found in the lower forms of life. With the development of the cerebrum, control of reflex action and the partial replacement of reflex action by voluntary action take place. For example, if we touch something hot, the natural reflex action is to withdraw from the heat source. If, however, we pick up a hot plate with our dinner on it, we can continue to hold the plate and put it down safely at the expense of burnt fingers: the reflex is inhibited. If we have been warned and expect the plate to be hot this control is more easily established.

In the case of pure reflex, when the action which is produced has no value – for example, knee jerk – there is still some inhibiting effect from the brain, and if the nerve path to and from the brain to muscle is dislodged by injury or disease above the anterior horn all the action is much more marked.

Actions which are in the first place voluntary become, in a sense, reflex: for example, standing is in the first place a voluntary action which is produced by the will. When we have learned to keep our balance on two feet we learn to do it by the sensations from the skin of our feet, and from muscles and joints and the sensory organs of balance, and we can stand without voluntary effort unless disease affects the sensory nerves.

ACTIVITY 2   **// ALLOW 5 MINUTES**

Identify the reflex actions which may occur at the different levels.

Commentary

You may have identified:

- spinal reflex

- reflexes occurring at the base of the brain – sneezing, coughing, vomiting

- reflexes occurring in the cerebrum and involving use of the association fibres of the brain.

4: The autonomic nervous system

The autonomic nervous system supplies nerves to all the internal organs of the body and blood vessels. It is the part of the nervous system which controls and regulates the activities of smooth muscle, cardiac muscle and certain glands. The autonomic nervous system functions almost entirely without conscious control, and is controlled by centres of the brain, in particular by the cerebral cortex, the hypothalamus and the medulla oblongata.

The autonomic nervous system is thought to be almost entirely motor, with its efferent axons transmitting impulses from the central nervous system to visceral effectors. There are, however, some afferent fibres. Disease may impair or destroy these fibres without causing pain, and any pain which does occur is to a large extent due to inflammation of the lining membrane of the cavity in which they lie.

The autonomic nervous system consists of two parts: the sympathetic and para-sympathetic systems. Many organs innervated by the autonomic nervous system receive visceral efferent neurones from both components of the autonomic nervous system. In the main, impulses from one division will cause the organs to 'switch on' or increase activity, whilst impulses from the other division will have the reverse effect.

Sympathetic nervous system

The sympathetic nervous system consists of a double chain of ganglia running down the trunk just in front of the vertebral column in the cervical, thoracic and lumbar regions. They receive nerves from the thoracic and upper lumbar regions of the spinal cord. The sympathetic nervous system gives rise to:

- nerves supplying the internal organs – visceral branches

- nerves running back to the spinal nerves – parietal branches.

These nerves supply the blood vessels, sweat and sebaceous glands, and the muscles which raise the hairs of the skin. In certain regions where there are many organs requiring a nerve supply, there are additional ganglia between the two chains, linked by nerves with the chains and with one another, and supplying nerves to neighbouring organs. These are called plexus. Behind the heart in the thoracic region is the cardiac plexus and just below the diaphragm is the solar plexus, where the stomach, liver, spleen, kidneys and pancreas are found.

Parasympathetic nervous system

This consists chiefly of the vagus nerve, which supplies branches to all organs of the thorax and abdomen, and also includes the branches from the third, fourth and ninth cranial nerves and nerves from the ganglia in the sacral region of the spinal column.

Functions of the autonomic nervous system

All internal organs have a double nerve supply and the two sets of nerves have in each case opposite actions, one stimulating and one inhibiting the action of the organs.

Sympathetic nerves have a stimulating effect on the heart and on the respiratory system, but an inhibiting effect on digestion. They improve circulation and cause dilation of the bronchial tubes, increasing our intake of oxygen; they inhibit the secretion of digestive juices throughout the alimentary canal, and inhibit peristaltic action in its wall. They are stimulated by strong emotion such as anger, fear and excitement. The sympathetic nervous system enables the body to respond physiologically to emotion.

Parasympathetic nerves have the opposite effect, stimulating the digestive system. The vagus nerve slows the heart, reducing circulation, and has an inhibitory effect on the respiratory system. These nerves are stimulated by pleasant emotions.

ACTIVITY 3	// ALLOW 20 MINUTES

The following questions test your knowledge of the contents of Sessions One to Four.

1   What is the name given to the cell and its fibre?

2   Name the connective tissue which binds the cells and fibres together.

3   Name the two types of fibre.

4   Name the two coats of the nerve sheath.

5   List the three functions of the myelin sheath.

6   Can fibres regrow?

7   What are the two types of efferent neurone called?

8   Name the neurone which runs between the afferent and efferent neurones.

9   What is the name given to the special neurones of the skin?

10   What is the name given to the transmission of messages between neurones?

11   What chemical substance must be present to allow transmission to take place?

12   Name the two electrical ions also present.

13   Name the two nervous systems.

14   List the five parts of the brain.

15   Name the four lobes of the hemispheres.

16   Identify four functions of the cerebral cortex.

17   Name the structure which joins the two hemispheres.

18   Which is outside on the spinal cord, grey or white matter?

19   Which is outside on the brain, grey or white matter?

20   Name the fifth and seventh cranial nerves.

21   How many pairs of spinal nerves are there?

22   Name the three nerves of the tracheal plexus.

23   Name the two branches of the sciatic nerve from the division above the knee.

24   Name the chief nerve of the parasympathetic nervous system.

25   Which nerves improve circulation and cause dilation of the bronchial tubes?

Commentary

1   Neurone.

2   Neuroglia.

3   Axon and dendrite.

4   Neurilemma and myelin sheath.

5   Protection, nutrition and insulation.

6   Yes.

7   Motor neurones and secretory neurones.

8   Association or connective neurones.

9   Unipolar neurones.

10   Synapse.

11   Acetylcholine.

12   Potassium and chloride.

13   Central and autonomic.

14   Cerebrum, midbrain, pons Varolii, medulla oblongata and cerebellum.

15   Frontal, parietal, temporal and occipital.

16   Motor, sensory, special senses and mental powers.

17   Corpus callosum.

18   White.

19   Grey.

20   Trigeminal and facial.

21   3l.

22   Radial, ulnar and median.

23   Popliteal and tibial.

24   Vagus nerve.

25   Sympathetic.

Before you move on to Session Five, check that you have achieved the objectives given at the beginning of this session and, if not, review the appropriate sections.

The human experience of pain

Introduction

In this session we discuss the human experience of pain. We review the history of pain, distinguish between acute and chronic pain, and discuss the modulation of pain.

Session objectives

When you have completed this session you should be able to:

● discuss the belief that pain is not a sensation but an emotion

● identify the different types of pain and their physiological background

● explain the functions of the two main types of nociceptor

● discuss the value of superficial electrical stimulus in the control of acute pain

● evaluate the stimulation of the brain and the spinal cord in the control of pain.

1: The history of pain

Aristotle, the Greek philosopher, believed that humans had five senses: sight, hearing, taste, smell and touch. He regarded pain not as a sensation but as an emotion, roughly opposite to the emotion of pleasure. Modern science, however, would disagree with this classification. Some scientists might consider pain to be a sensation somewhat similar to the sensation of touch. Aristotle could be considered partially correct in considering pain to be an emotion, as evidence suggests that our individual perception of pain varies with mood, attitude towards pain and a host of other psychological variables.

ACTIVITY 1 // ALLOW 10 MINUTES

Recall two occasions when you experienced pain, and identify any other factors occurring at the same time which may have contributed to, or detracted from, the degree of pain you experienced.

Commentary

Obviously your experiences will be unique to you, but you may have found that the pain related to an injury while playing a competitive sport was modified by the excitement of the game. On the other hand, a headache experienced when awakening might have felt worse if you knew that a stressful day at work was ahead.

Although we have all experienced pain, it remains a uniquely personal experience. Your experience of toothache will be different from someone else's, although if someone says that he or she is suffering from toothache you will be able to relate to that experience through memories of your own pain.

This variability in pain experience between individuals and in the same individual at different times and under different circumstances would suggest that there are complex neural mechanisms involving pain perception and the interpretation of pain.

ACTIVITY 2 // ALLOW 30 MINUTES

If you had to differentiate between acute and chronic pain, how would you describe acute pain?

Once you have written your thoughts down, you should read *Resource 3, Pathophysiology of acute pain*, from the *Resources Section*.

Commentary

The section below will assist you in differentiating between various pain classifications.

2: Types of pain

There are several different kinds of pain, caused by different mechanisms occurring at the site of the injury. Clinical experience suggests that each different kind of pain requires different treatment or combinations of treatments to produce relief.

Acute, sharp, intense pain associated with an immediate injury is usually considered to be important in survival terms. Unpleasant severe pain often leads to a rapid reflex response, removing part or all of the body from the damaging stimulus. For example, fast spinal reflexes, discussed in Session Four, will cause the immediate removal of a hand or finger which comes into contact with a hot surface. This type of reflex response is so fast that it is not until a second or two afterwards that the brain registers that the hand has been removed from the source of the pain.

The situation with chronic pain is different. Depending on the injury there may be some survival value associated with the chronic pain. For example, if a person sprains his or her ankle there will be survival value lasting for a few days to ensure that the joint is immobilised to enable healing to commence. The chronic pain may be present for some time while tissues are inflamed. When prolonged and severe pain results from chronic tissue pathology, it can have major adverse effects on both the quality and duration of life. Such chronic pain represents a serious problem for the patient and is very difficult to treat.

Within this session we have identified that there are two types of pain – acute and chronic – and that there can be an overlap of both as identified in the example of a sprained ankle. It is thought that different types of pain are mediated by different nociceptors which in turn are associated with different nerve fibres that carry the sensory information back to the spinal cord. Nociceptors are specialised receptors closely associated with particular sensory nerves which are located in the neural membranes of the terminal fibres of the primary sensory neurones.

ACTIVITY 3	// ALLOW 5 MINUTES

Name the two main types of nociceptor involved in the perception of pain.

Commentary

The two main types of nociceptor are:

- mechano-nociceptors

- polymodal nociceptors.

Mechano-nociceptors are only activated by intense mechanical pressure such as pinching. This type of receptor is associated with sensory nerve fibres known as AΩ fibres, which are thinly myelinated fast-conducting fibres. These receptors do not respond to chemical mediators, which are normally released during tissue damage or inflammation. They are activated by low-intensity mechanical stimuli such as touch, gentle pressure or brushing.

Polymodal nociceptors respond to a variety of noxious stimuli, including pressure and heat, as well as to a wide range of chemical mediators released from cells during tissue damage or inflammation. The nerve fibres associated with the polymodal receptors are the C fibres, which are unmyelinated and which conduct impulses much slower than the AΩ fibres. The C fibres carry high-intensity stimulation that gives the sensation of burning, powerful pressure or painful pinching.

Both types of fibre are widely distributed in the skin as well as in most internal organs and tissues.

3: Modulation of pain

Humans and other animals instinctively rub or lick small wounds or injuries to reduce the sensation of pain. It should therefore be possible to modify pain perception by increasing input from some other form of sensory input – a non-drug method of modulating the pain response.

ACTIVITY 4 // ALLOW 15 MINUTES

Read *Resource 4* from the *Resources Section* to recap on the *Management of the individual with pain* and make brief notes for yourself.

Commentary

Depending upon how long ago you began your career you may remember the seminal work of Melzack and Wall in 1965. At that time theirs was considered to be a major step forward towards our understanding of pain and pain pathways. Since that time their theory has been challenged, modified and expanded. It is well worth reading about.

ACTIVITY 5 // ALLOW 5 MINUTES

From your own experience, identify the type of patients in pain who may benefit from the use of transcutaneous electrical nerve stimulation (TENS) and those who may not.

Commentary

We discuss the use of transcutaneous electrical nerve stimulation below.

The use of superficial electrical stimulation to control pain

Stimulation of the sensory nerve endings in superficial nerves can be achieved by applying electrodes to the skin. This stimulates mechano-receptors which have a lower threshold than nociceptive fibres, and it is possible to evoke electrical responses without the sensation of pain. This technique is termed transcutaneous electrical nerve stimulation (TENS). This form of relief from pain lasts longer than the period of electrical stimulation and in some patients periods of TENS stimulation of about l5 minutes will produce pain relief lasting for several hours. About 60 per cent of patients can obtain relief from acute pain with TENS. Unfortunately, the technique is less effective in patients with chronic pain.

Direct stimulation of the brain and spinal cord to control pain

Researchers have known that electrical stimulation of the central nervous system in animals can cause severe pain and many no longer use animals in this way. However, in the last 30 to 40 years it has been discovered that stimulation of certain regions within the spinal cord and brain produces profound analgesia and the total absence of pain sensation.

In humans, stimulation of the grey matter surrounding the third ventricle – in particular the peri-ventricular grey matter – almost totally abolishes any sensation of pain, no matter how severe the pain was before the electrodes were implanted.

It is interesting to note that some patients do not lose their sensitivity to other sensory information and that they can still respond to touch, pressure and temperature; they just do not feel pain. This is called stimulation-produced analgesia, and in selected patients can provide an effective means of pain control. In some patients electrodes can be implanted and the devices controlled by the patient, who can alter the frequency and duration of stimulation to give maximum relief from pain.

Animal experiments investigating the mechanisms involved in stimulation-produced analgesia demonstrated that the analgesia produced by electrical stimulation of the central nervous system was reversed by the same drugs that were marketed to reverse the analgesic effects of morphine. This observation gave rise to the hypothesis that certain neurones in the brain and the spinal cord synthesise and release a natural morphine-like substance that serves, as a neurotransmitter, which acts upon inhibiting neurones to modify our perception of pain. It is these naturally occurring analgesic systems which we will consider in the next session.

Before you move on to Session Six, check that you have achieved the objectives given at the beginning of this session and, if not, review the appropriate sections.

Natural analgesic systems

Introduction

In this session we look at the natural analgesic systems of the human body. We start by discussing the endogenous opioid systems of the body and their role in controlling pain. We then go on to consider how acupuncture draws upon these systems to control pain. We also discuss the issues of referred pain and projected or phantom pain.

Session objectives

When you have completed this session you should be able to:

- describe the endogenous opioid system

- explain the role of the endogenous opioid system in the control of pain

- examine the role of acupuncture in pain control

- explain the pathophysiology of referred pain

- discuss the phenomenon of phantom or projected pain.

1: The endogenous opioid systems

In the previous session we saw that research demonstrated that electrical stimulation of the brain produced analgesia. The same researchers went on to establish that stimulation of descending nerve tracts in the spinal cord inhibited the generation of action potentials in the nociceptive neurones in the laminae of the dorsal root of the spinal cord. They also established that the injection of low concentrations of morphine into the same regions of the brain as those electrically stimulated produced profound and long-lasting analgesia. These studies demonstrated that:

- the sites where morphine exerted its analgesic action were in the central nervous system

- the sites at which morphine acted were the same sites that produced analgesia when stimulated electrically.

In the early 1970s, two scientific advances were made that have greatly increased the knowledge base of how neuronal pathways in the central nervous system act to modify our perception of pain.

- Snyder and Pet (in 1973) demonstrated that the brain contains receptors that selectively combine with morphine and related drugs

- Hughes and Kosterlitz (in 1975) demonstrated that the brain contains small peptide molecules which act as opioids (morphine-like drugs).

It is known that there are three classes of endogenous (naturally occurring) opioid found in the central nervous system:

- enkephalins

- endorphins

- dynorphins.

Each of these three classes of endogenous opioid peptides derives from separate genes, and each brings about analgesia. However, the enkephalins and a sub-division of the endorphins known as B-endorphins are more potent than the dynorphins.

The physiological importance of these endogenous opioid peptides can be summarised as follows:

- they are located in the central nervous system in the areas associated with the processing or modulation of nociception

- they act as neurotransmitters and are located in nerve endings

- the neurones containing enkephalin and dynorphins are concentrated in the grey matter of the dorsal horn of the spinal cord, in particular in laminae I and II

- B-endorphins are concentrated in the hypothalamus and the grey matter surrounding the third ventricle

- morphine and related drugs bind to three sub-types of opiate receptor: mu, delta and kappa

- the enkephalins bind to and activate the mu and delta sub-types

- the dynorphins activate the kappa receptors.

You should note that the analgesic effect of morphine and endogenous opioid peptides is reversed by morphine antagonists such as naloxone.

The control of pain by the endogenous opioid systems

ACTIVITY 1   **// ALLOW 10 MINUTES**

Make notes on the possible significance of the excitatory neurones from the cerebral cortex and hypothalamus impinging upon the periaqueductal grey matter.

Commentary

The periaqueductal grey matter of the midbrain contains a high concentration of opioid receptors which, when stimulated electrically, produce profound analgesia. As the cerebral cortex is concerned with conscious thought and the hypothalamus is involved in the expression of emotion, it is reasonable to suggest that excitatory neurones arising from the areas of the brain and forming synapses in the periaqueductal grey matter are related to the modulation by conscious will power and by emotion.

The periaqueductal grey matter contains both a high concentration of opiate receptors and opioid peptides. Neurones from this grey matter make excitatory connections with neurones located in the medulla oblongata. Axons from the medulla oblongata project down the spinal cord in the descending spinal pathways to form synapses in the dorsal horn of the spinal cord.

As has previously been identified, the laminae of the dorsal horn are very rich in neuronal connections, receiving inputs from many sensory neurones. They are also rich in a variety of neurotransmitters present at the different synapses. Not only do neurones contain opioid peptides such as enkephalins and dynorphins; they also contain amide transmitters such as noradrenaline, acetylcholine and 5-hydroxytryptamine, and amino acid transmitters such as glutamine and glycerine, and the peptide transmitter, Substance P.

ACTIVITY 2   **// ALLOW 15 MINUTES**

The chemistry of the opioid system is quite complex. Think of an example of how endorphins could be explained to a colleague, client or relative.

Commentary

It is known and accepted that the brain can influence the perception of pain. If certain areas of the brain and spinal cord are stimulated electrically, feelings of pain can be abolished. The perception of pain can be altered by other factors. For example, emotions such as fear can reduce the perception of pain.

Scientists have identified three types of peptide neurotransmitter – endorphins, enkephalins and dynorphins – which are all naturally occurring analgesic transmitters which act upon receptors to block transmission across synapses in the ascending nociceptive pathways and so reduce the amount of nociceptive sensory information reaching the brain. These neurotransmitters are also released from nerve terminals located on neurones in the descending neuronal pathway. Morphine and morphine-like analgesic drugs exert their effect by stimulating the same receptors as do these natural opioid peptides.

2: Acupuncture – an example of opioid pain control

ACTIVITY 3 // ALLOW 15 MINUTES

Before continuing, you should first make short notes on what you understand about how acupuncture can be used to relieve pain. Once you have done this you should read *Resource 5*.

Commentary

We will now discuss acupuncture.

Acupuncture was developed many centuries ago in China as a method of pain control, and is still used throughout the world today. Acupuncture involves placing fine needles in certain defined areas of the skin in an attempt to attain analgesia in specific parts of the body. Clinical evidence indicates that acupuncture is effective in about 50 per cent of patients who are about to undergo minor surgery or other procedures with transient pain. There is little research available on the mode of action of the acupuncture procedure but in both humans and animals the use of acupuncture needles increases the release of endorphins into the cerebrospinal fluid. It has also been discovered that in humans the analgesic effect of acupuncture is blocked by an injection of naloxone, a drug known to block the effect of endorphins at the opioid receptors.

There is neither the time nor the space within this unit to explore other therapeutic approaches to pain control. However, once you have completed this unit you may wish to explore areas such as:

● hypnosis

- therapeutic massage

- homeopathy

- Bach flowers

- chiropractic

- cognitive behavioural therapy.

3: Referred pain

Referred pain is a peculiar aspect of pain which arises in a deep tissue or organ, but is experienced as arising in some superficial tissue or organ.

ACTIVITY 4	ALLOW 5 MINUTES

From you own professional or personal experience list a few examples of referred pain.

Commentary

One of the most commonly known examples is the pain resulting from myocardial ischaemia, which is perceived as coming from the superficial muscle of the left shoulder or arm and not only from the regions of the heart. Other examples include pain from an infection of the kidney tissue, not felt in the back over the kidney but perceived as coming from the groin. Or the intestinal pain produced by an inflammation of the appendix which is perceived as coming from the superficial muscles along the mid-line of the abdomen when in fact the appendix is situated in the right inguinal fossa.

Referred pain can be explained if one revisits the embryonic origin of the nerve supply. For example, the heart first develops in the head/neck region of the embryo and so it receives its nerve supply from the cervical segments of the developing spinal cord. Later, when the heart migrates to its position in the chest, it takes the nerve supply with it, retaining its links with the cervical sections of the cord. In the adult, the shoulders and arms also receive their nerve supply from a similar area of the cord (lamina V). It is because of this embryonic link that the visceral (heart) and the somatic (shoulder/arm) pain fibres share a common pathway to the sensory cortex through their 'address' in lamina V. This explains why the pain from myocardial ischaemia is experienced as pain which radiates into the left arm and/or shoulder.

In many clinical cases the anatomical site of referred pain is so constant in its location that it is a valuable aid to early diagnosis.

4: Projected or phantom pain

It could be argued that loss or damage to the peripheral sensory neurones which carry the nerve impulses from the nociceptors to the spinal cord, as would occur through injury or amputation, would impair pain sensations and, indeed, this is often the case. However, severe pain can arise spontaneously in the absence of stimulation of the nociceptors. This type of pain is termed neuropathic pain and results from damage or disease of the peripheral sensory nerves following surgery, traumatic injury or tumour infiltration. Neuropathic pain is exceedingly difficult to treat and is a major clinical problem in providing pain relief.

Amputees often experience sensations that appear to come from the severed limb. This is called the 'phantom limb sensation', or phantom pain, and presumably results from activation of the sensory pathway either at the site of the amputation – that is, damaged or regenerated nerve endings – or within the central nervous system. In some patients these phantom experiences present as severe pain which is very difficult to control, as is often the case in amputation following emergency surgery rather than planned surgery.

Before you move on to Session Seven, check that you have achieved the objectives given at the beginning of this session and, if not, review the appropriate sections.

The development of chronic pain

Introduction

In this session we look at the development of chronic pain. We start by looking at how different types of pain are transmitted: in particular, we look at the role played by peripheral sensitisation and hyperalgesia in transmitting chronic pain. We then consider the role of a range of chemical mediators in transmitting pain. Next, we look at drugs that relieve pain by sensitising the nociceptors. Finally, we consider the issue of central sensitisation to pain, and consider the problem of peripheral nerve damage.

Session objectives

When you have completed this session you should be able to:

● distinguish between the three categories of pain

● explain the mechanisms which give rise to chronic pain

● discuss the concepts of hyperalgesia and secondary hyperalgesia

● discuss the notion of 'wind-up' as a major feature of chronic pain.

1: Transmission of types of pain

As discussed earlier, the sharp intense pain we feel when standing on something sharp or twisting an ankle are examples of protective pain which warns us of something dangerous in the environment that we should avoid. However, if we have twisted our ankle badly then that sharp protective pain is rapidly replaced by a more diffuse, throbbing pain that spreads along the foot and leg, and triggers the emotion of distress or fear. We possibly know from experience that this pain is going to be with us for some time and that it is going to be very unpleasant if we attempt to walk on the damaged foot.

The relative speed of delivery of different types of pain does not just depend on the different nociceptive fibres involved, but also on what happens to the pain pathways when they reach the central nervous system. We previously identified that the nociceptive impulses enter through the dorsal root of the spinal cord and then ascend the spinal cord through specialised nerve tracts to the base of the brain. The majority of these ascending spinal tracts form their first synapse in the thalamus. However, a small proportion of the fibres that carry information about pain do not synapse in the thalamus but pass directly to the cerebellum. It is the information transmitted along these fibres directly to the sensory cortex that allows the brain to localise the site of pain, rather than information that has been slightly distorted by passing through one or more synapses in the thalamus.

The majority of the nociceptive impulses, especially those transmitted by the C fibres, synapse in the thalamus. In the thalamus the nociceptive neurones can form numerous synapses with other nerve fibres. These transmit the nociceptive information not only to the cerebral cortex but also to other areas of the brain, such as the hypothalamus, which have important influences both over emotional reactions and the control of internal systems such as heart rate, blood pressure and respiration. This transmission has important consequences both for our perception and experience of pain.

The larger number of synapses in the thalamus distorts the information so it can no longer be projected forward on to discrete areas of the sensory cortex. This means that we cannot localise the pain to a precise anatomical location but rather perceive it as a dull aching pain involving quite large areas of the body. Secondly, the transmission of information to other areas of the brain aggravates nerve tracts that give rise to emotional perceptions associated with pain, including the intense, unpleasant physical symptoms associated with chronic pain.

ACTIVITY 1 // ALLOW 5 MINUTES

List the main bodily sensations you think can be associated with severe diffuse pain. (One example would be sweating.)

Commentary

The physical symptoms that accompany severe pain can be very variable. However, it is common to see one or more of the following:

● sweating

● nausea

● an alteration of blood pressure

● a general reduction in skeletal muscle tone.

ACTIVITY 2 // ALLOW 15 MINUTES

Describe the three major forms of pain.

Commentary

The first is protective pain, of the type associated with the withdrawal reflex. This acts as an immediate warning of danger or tissue damage and provides the necessary information to allow the central nervous system to make an immediate response.

The second is the type of pain experienced if the stimulus that produces the protective pain response is severe enough to lead to tissue damage: for example, breaking a limb. The immediate sharp pain associated with the trauma of the injury rapidly fades and is replaced by a deep developing pain that is diffuse around the site of the injury. This may be accompanied by a reflex action affecting the autonomic nervous system, producing a feeling of dizziness or nausea. This type of pain has a survival role in that it makes the injured person keep the limb still in order to prevent further tissue damage and promote healing. The dull aching pain will eventually go away as the bone and the surrounding tissues heal and recover from the injury. It may be some weeks, however, before the injured site is completely pain-free. Continued pain ensures the injured individual does not apply excessive pressure or activity to the injured part until healing has occurred.

The third type of pain is more difficult to treat and exists when the tissues do not recover from injury but are subjected to continual and chronic damage. This type of pain is known as chronic pain and although often associated with the terminal stage of some forms of cancer is also present in other clinical conditions that are not necessarily terminal, for example the pain associated with rheumatoid arthritis.

Having looked at the first and second types of pain in previous sessions, it is now time to look at the third type – chronic pain – in some detail. Chronic pain develops when both the sensory neurones and nociceptors become extra sensitive, due to prolonged exposure to inflammatory mediators released during chronic tissue inflammation.

There are two interrelated mechanisms which contribute to the development of this sensitivity.

Peripheral sensitivity occurs when the receptors of the site of the injury become more sensitive to stimulation by inflammatory mediators.

Central sensitivity occurs when chronic pain is severe and lasts for sufficient time to alter the nature of neurotransmission in the spinal cord. When this happens the spinal neurones become abnormally sensitive to impulses arising from the nociceptors. This increases the amount of information that is transmitted upwards to the brain which in turn interprets the signals as enhanced pain.

Peripheral sensitisation

Unlike other sensory receptors, nociceptors do not show adaptation when exposed to a constant stimulus. Indeed, the opposite occurs and if tissue damage is severe and prolonged the nociceptors increase in sensitivity. When peripheral tissues are damaged they release a number of chemical mediators either from the damaged cells or from specialised inflammatory cells. These mediators sensitise the nociceptors and this results in an increase in nerve impulse traffic along the sensory neurones to the spinal cord leading to an enhancement of the sensation of pain. This increase in the perception of pain results from two different, but related, changes that occur in the sensitivity of the nociceptors to the chemical mediators. These changes are important in the development of chronic pain.

Hyperalgesia

In hyperalgesia the chemicals mediating pain lower the threshold of the nociceptor to stimulation. This means that not only do the nociceptors respond to lower concentrations of the chemical mediator but nociceptors distant from the original site of damage are also sensitised, leading to the sensation of pain spreading over a wider area. The increased sensitivity of the nociceptors to the pain mediators results in increased formation and frequency of action potentials travelling along the sensory neurones to the spinal cord and then to the brain.

ACTIVITY 3 // ALLOW 5 MINUTES

Why do you think the perception of pain increases following an increase in the sensitivity of the nociceptors to pain mediators?

Commentary

A consequence of the lowering of the nociceptors' threshold of sensitivity is that a previously mild stimulus which provoked only a few action potentials in the sensory nerves will now provoke rapid sequences of action potentials. The increase in the number of action potentials arriving at the spinal cord will be interpreted by the central nervous system as an increase in the severity of the pain.

Another consequence of hyperalgesia is that previously innocuous stimuli that did not trigger a response may now cause severe pain. For example, a light touch to the skin close to the inflamed area may be perceived as severe pain. Another example is the throbbing sensation that is common in inflamed tissue. This is a result of the movement of blood through small arteries which would normally not be noticed because the vibrations of the blood vessels are usually insufficient to trigger the nociceptors.

Sensitisation – secondary hyperalgesia

This is similar to hyperalgesia but is more common in situations where there is continuing tissue inflammation and damage resulting in the release of a diverse variety of chemical mediators. Increased sensitivity occurs in all types of nociceptor, as well as in receptors associated with other sensations such as touch and pressure. This involvement of different types of sensory receptor combined with the large number of chemical mediators involved in producing the increased sensitivity complicates the treatment of chronic pain in those patients where sensitisation has occurred.

2: Chemical mediators and the sensitisation of nociceptors

When tissues are damaged, the damaged cells release their intracellular chemicals such as potassium and also a large number of enzymes. The activation of these enzymes in the extracellular space generates the formation of new chemicals that act as mediators of the inflammatory response. The components that are produced as a result of tissue damage act at the terminal of the sensory neurones, either to decrease the stimulation threshold of the nociceptors to other pain mediators, or to activate the nociceptors directly to generate action potentials.

A practical example of this would be when a person grazes the knee when falling. When this happens there is damage to the skin and the underlying layers of tissue. The damaged cells either release chemicals (such as potassium) or enzymes that are activated when released and which in turn produce additional chemical mediators such as bradykinin which generates hypersensitivity in the immediate vicinity of the injured site. Many of these chemical mediators do not diffuse very far through the tissues, so peripheral sensitivity is restricted to close to the site of the injury.

When the damaged area is small, such as in a graze, then the pain and swelling associated with the damage will be limited to a small area. However, in a developing disease, such as a growing tumour, more and more tissue damage occurs leading to greater sensitisation of nociceptors over wide areas of the body.

Chemicals released from damaged tissues which activate or sensitise nociceptors

Table 1 summarises the effect of chemicals released from a variety of sources.

Chemical	Source	Effect
Histamine	Healthy cells	Activate
Prostaglandins	Damaged cells	Sensitise
Bradykinin	Plasma proteins	Activate
Substance P	Primary afferent neurones	Sensitise
Potassium	Damaged cells	Activate
5-hydroxytriptamine	Blood platelets	Activate

Table 1: Effects of chemicals

Histamine

Histamine is stored in special inflammatory cells called mast cells, and is released when the mast cells are damaged or activated. Histamine is commonly released during inflammatory reactions triggered by the immune response, such as those which occur in hay fever and asthma. A major role for the released histamine is to contribute to the inflammatory swelling by increasing the permeability of the capillaries to blood plasma, allowing both water and some molecular weight plasma proteins to escape into the extracellular space. Histamine also stimulates the polymodal nociceptors directly and if injected under the skin produces an intense sensation of burning pain.

Prostaglandins

All cells contain a class of enzymes called the phospholipases. These enzymes are normally present in an inactive form but are activated when the cells are damaged. A major role of the phospholipases is to release an unsaturated fatty acid – arachidonic acid – from the phospholipids of the cell membrane. The released arachidonic acid is immediately acted upon by another enzyme, cyclo-oxygenase. The cyclo-oxygenase converts the arachidonic acid into two classes of chemical mediators, the prostaglandins and the leukotrienes. Members of both families are important chemical mediators in pain and inflammation. They produce hyperalgesia and sensitise nociceptors to all other direct stimulants. The powerful pain-relieving and anti-inflammatory drugs such as aspirin and other non-steroidal anti-inflammatory drugs inhibit the action of the enzyme cyclo-oxygenase and so prevent the formation of the prostaglandins.

ACTIVITY 4 // **ALLOW 15 MINUTES**

In light of the above description of the action of prostaglandins, how do you think that aspirin reduces pain?

Commentary

By inhibiting the enzyme cyclo-oxygenase aspirin prevents it from converting arachidonic acid into the chemical mediator prostaglandin. This prevents the prostaglandins from producing hyperalgesia and causing sensitisation of the nociceptors to other mediators released.

Aspirin is very effective in reducing pain associated with inflammation such as after removal of a tooth or in arthritis. It is, however, less effective in reducing pain in non-inflamed tissue such as bone pain.

Bradykinin

During inflammation and tissue damage, plasma proteins and occasionally blood cells will leak through the capillary wall to produce swelling and oedema. Bradykinin is a polypeptide chemical mediator produced from a plasma protein called kininogen by the enzyme kallikrien, which is activated in areas of damaged cells during the development of inflammation.

Bradykinin is one of the most active pain-producing agents known. It not only stimulates both AΩ and C nociceptors to increase the rate of production of action; it also stimulates the release of prostaglandins from nearby tissues. The prostaglandins further increase the sensitivity of the nociceptors not only to bradykinin but also to stimulate agents, such as potassium released from damaged cells and histamine released from mast cells.

There is also evidence that during chronic inflammation a new type of bradykinin receptor acts upon the nociceptive nerves. The appearance of the additional bradykinin receptor may be related to the development of the long-lasting sensitivity of the nociceptors that is a characteristic of severe chronic pain and which makes it so difficult to treat.

Substance P

In chronic pain the prolonged exposure to chemical mediators and the increase in nerve impulse traffic brings about changes in the expression of genes present in the cell bodies of the nociceptive neurones. One of the changes is that genes which control the synthesis of biologically active peptides are activated so that the sensory neurones now synthesise and release more neurotransmitters and also synthesise and release 'new' neurotransmitters such as Substance P. Substance P released from the nerve endings of sensory neurones diffuses away from the original site of inflammation and activates neighbouring nociceptive nerve endings which were not involved in the original injury. This is one of the mechanisms by which the area of painful sensation can spread widely through an organ or tissue during progressive tissue damage.

Substance P is more than just an important mediator in the sensitisation of nociceptors at peripheral sites of damage. Increased synthesis of Substance P results in its release at synapses that the sensory neurone makes with the interneurones within the laminae of the spinal cord, so increasing sensitisation of nociceptors.

3: Drugs that relieve chronic pain by influencing nociceptors

The development of chronic pain is a complex process involving both chemical mediators and a change in the genetic control of the neurotransmitter function of the neurones that make up nociceptive pathways. Most chronic pain develops during some form of inflammation, whether this results from the infiltration of tissue by malignant growth, neuropathology or as the result of infection. It is during this inflammatory response and resulting tissue damage that nociceptors become sensitised and activated by the chemicals released from damaged cells or formed by the activation of enzymes. These complex interactions make it difficult, if not impossible, to develop one drug that will be clinically useful in relieving the symptoms of all types of chronic pain.

Chronic pain is experienced differently from other forms of pain. The psychological and emotional overlay that accompanies the experience of severe chronic pain adds to the complexity of treating individual patients. The importance of psychological factors in the management of chronic pain is underlined by the observation that many drugs that are very potent analgesics in laboratory tests are not acceptable to patients for the treatment of chronic pain because the pharmacological profile of the drug does not include euphoric or sedative effects on the central nervous system. However, work continues to develop more effective painkillers and to find more effective ways of using the existing range of drugs, based upon our increasing understanding of nociceptive mechanisms and the interactions between the various chemical mediators.

ACTIVITY 5   // ALLOW 20 MINUTES

Make a list of possible sites of action for new drugs which could be useful in reducing peripheral sensitisation in chronic pain.

Commentary

The common mediator in producing both sensitisation of the nociceptors and the release of stimulating mediators is Substance P. If a drug could be developed that could prevent the synthesis and release of Substance P then the sensitisation and activation of the nociceptors by the other chemical mediators would be prevented or reduced.

It may be possible to develop a receptor-blocking drug for Substance P which would prevent it from releasing both bradykinin and histamine, and perhaps also prevent the direct sensitisation of the nociceptors by Substance P.

Some pain relief can also be obtained by preventing the action of other chemical mediators such as bradykinin, prostaglandins and perhaps histamine. Aspirin acts at this level to prevent the formation of prostaglandins.

The long-term consequences of chronic inflammatory pain are, however, more complex than simple alteration in the threshold of excitability for peripheral nociceptors. In addition to altering the activity of the peripheral nociceptors, many of the chemical messengers released from tissue cells during inflammation have more profound effects on the sensory neurones. They penetrate into the nerve endings of the sensory neurone and are transported along the axon to the neurone by axoplasmic flow. When these chemical messengers reach the cell body in the dorsal root of the spinal cord, they then influence the expression of genes in the cell nucleus so that the neurone synthesises new and unexpected chemical messengers. These, in turn, can contribute to the development of chronic pain by altering the characteristics of synaptic transmission at the interneurones in the spinal cord.

4: Central sensitisation

When patients develop a disease that results in chronic intractable pain their sensitivity to pain increases and their tolerance of it decreases. Once this sensitisation becomes established the management of the patient's pain becomes more difficult as increasingly large doses of the most potent analgesics will be required to control the pain. This aggressive treatment can then lead to significant increases of side effects produced by the analgesics which might mitigate against the better pain control achieved by using these higher drug doses.

So far in this session we have looked at the mechanisms underlying the phenomenon of the nociceptors' increased sensitivity to pain by considering the role played by peripheral mediators such as Substance P and the prostaglandins. We are now beginning to learn something of the mechanisms of increased sensitivity to pain that arises in the central nervous system, especially in the spinal cord. This area is another important one which needs to be considered when planning drug therapy for patients with chronic pain.

The phenomenon of increased sensitivity to pain resulting from changes in the properties of nociceptor neurones in the spinal cord is referred to by a number of names. We will use the term 'wind-up' because that describes what happens at the synapses in the spinal cord. The effect of untreated chronic pain on the synaptic activity of the spinal nociceptive neurones is to increase the amount of impulse traffic flowing through the synapse. This effect is similar to winding up a mechanical toy so it will go faster and faster.

ACTIVITY 6	// ALLOW 10 MINUTES

We have considered the actions of inflammatory mediators on the peripheral nociceptors. Some of these points are relevant to the understanding of spinal 'wind-up'. By way of revision you should fill in the missing words in the following paragraph.

'Following tissue injury and inflammation a number of _____ _____ (1) such as Substance P, prostaglandins, histamine and K+ are released. These mediators act at the _____ (2) to stimulate them directly, or increase their _____ (3) (lower the threshold) to stimulants, or both. This then produces hyperalgesia where the _____ (4) become very sensitive to any form of activating stimuli. The increased activation of the nociceptor results in an increase in _____ _____ (5) along the sensory neurone to the spinal cord. From here the impulses are projected up the _____ _____ _____ (6) to the _____ _____ __ ___ _____ (7). The increase in impulse traffic resulting from the _____ __ ___ _____ (8) is interpreted by the higher centres of the brain as an _____ (9) experience of the sensation of pain.'

Commentary

(1) chemical mediators (2) nociceptors (3) sensitivity (4) nociceptors (5) impulse traffic (6) ascending spinal tracts (7) higher centres of the brain (8) sensitisation of the nociceptors (9) increased.

In addition to the above, the increase in impulse traffic from the sensitised nociceptors also has effects on synaptic transmissions in the spinal cord and perhaps other nociceptive pathways higher up the central nervous system. During the development of chronic pain the nociceptive network undergoes adaptation by changes occurring in the role and function of neurotransmitters at the synapses and in the number of receptors present at the synapse.

Synthesis of neurotransmitters in sensory neurones

If we were to electrically stimulate the axons of the $A\underline{\Omega}$ and C sensory fibres in order to simulate pain, and then measure the release of neurotransmitters in the spinal cord, we would find that not one but several neurotransmitters are released in the dorsal horn of the spinal cord. Thus, multiplicity of neurotransmitters at a single synapse appears to be related to the modulation of the activity of the neural networks by the interneurones. The different neurotransmitters are used in central synaptic transmission by being released at differential rates that depend upon the frequency of nerve action potentials. Amongst these many neurotransmitters there is a mixture of excitatory and inhibitory neurotransmitters, and the mutual potentiation or inhibition provided by this arrangement gives an additional mechanism for fine control of synaptic transmission. It is easy to visualise a system operating at the synapse where the amount and type of neurotransmitter released will be continually varied according to the intensity of the sensory input reaching the synapse.

An important excitatory neurotransmitter at sensory synapses in the spinal cord appears to be the excitatory amino acid, glutamate. The same neurones also release other neuropeptide neurotransmitters such as Substance P and neurokinin. The importance of these excitatory transmitters in the propagation of nociceptive information is that it is the function of the enkephalin-containing interneurones in the spinal cord to inhibit the release of glutamate, Substance P and other excitatory transmitters from the terminal axons of the nociceptive neurones, and so prevent the passages of pain impulses reaching the brain.

During the development of chronic pain there is a time-dependent increase in the synthesis of Substance P (and perhaps the other transmitters) so that more Substance P is being released from the nociceptive neurone. The effect of Substance P at the synapse is not to act as a transmitter but to increase the number of receptors for the excitatory amino acids such as glutamate. This leads to increased effectiveness of glutamate as an excitatory transmitter and reduces the effectiveness of the enkephalins in preventing or reducing the passage of pain impulses across the synapse. The result is that more impulses pass to the ascending spinal neurone and up to the higher centres of the brain, increasing a person's experience and perception of pain.

Current treatment strategy for the prevention or reversal of 'wind-up' is to reduce impulse traffic between the nociceptive axon and the projection neurone by giving high doses of opiate drugs to the patient until the pain has completely disappeared, then reducing the dose of drugs to the minimum to keep the person pain-free.

5: Neuropathic pain

Neuropathic pain is another type of chronic pain that results from damage to the peripheral nerves. Following peripheral nerve damage, in which there is intensive damage to the axons but the cell bodies in the spinal cord remain intact, the nerves grow new neurones. However, some of the axons of these new neurones make the wrong connections. In the laminae of the spinal cord, for example, some 'normal' sensory neurones for touch might make connections with interneurones that normally receive input from nociceptors. This leads to the agonising sensitivity people with some forms of nerve damage have to light touch. This abnormal rewiring in the spinal cord also appears to contribute to the severity of neuropathic pain and its resistance to all forms of conventional treatment.

To summarise the information introduced in this session, we now know that there are two mechanisms which are primarily involved in the development of chronic pain.

● Peripheral mechanisms, which involve chemical messengers released as a result of tissue damage and inflammation, and which sensitise nociceptors and lower their stimulation threshold.

● A central mechanism, which involves the synapses in the grey matter of the spinal cord. The increased release of neurotransmitters and the formation of new transmitters through altered gene expression facilitate the increased passage of impulses across the synapse.

The increase in sensory information reaching the central nervous system is interpreted as chronic and severe pain.

ACTIVITY 7 // **ALLOW 10 MINUTES**

From your past nursing experience relate this new information to a patient you have nursed.

Commentary

Your response to this activity will depend on your nursing experience.

Before you move on to Session Eight, check that you have achieved the objectives given at the beginning of this session and, if not, review the appropriate sections.

The pharmacology of pain control

Introduction

In this session we look at the pharmacology of pain control. We start by defining the most important terms used in the session, then go on to discuss an important group of drugs – the non-steroidal anti-inflammatory drugs or NSAIDs. We consider the mechanisms of NSAIDs, their therapeutic uses and some of the side effects which can be associated with them. Next, we discuss the use of opioids: how they work, their pharmacological properties, their effects, their therapeutic use and the problems of tolerance, withdrawal and dependence. Finally, we consider the use of some other drugs to relieve pain.

Session objectives

When you have completed this session you should be able to:

● identify the three main groups of analgesic drugs

● explain the main functions of non-opioid drugs

● explain the main mechanisms of opioid drugs

● discuss the use of adjutant drugs.

1: Definitions

The role of the nurse as a member of the multi-disciplinary team is to work with the patient to devise a drug regime which reduces the patient's perception of pain to a minimum. The regime should support the patient's recovery and also maintain the mental and emotional well-being of the patient in chronic or terminal pain.

The choice of drugs available to alleviate pain is very wide.

ACTIVITY 1   **// ALLOW 5 MINUTES**

What factors need to be considered when determining a drug regime for patients suffering with chronic pain?

Commentary

The selection of a particular class of drugs to alleviate pain in a particular patient or condition is governed by a number of factors, including:

- the severity of the pain

- the expected duration of the pain – whether it is acute short-term pain seen after surgery or an accident, or chronic pain

- the patient's previous response to analgesic drugs, particularly the individual's tolerance to side effects

- the patient's emotional state and attitude to the cause of pain – this can be of paramount importance in chronic pain or the pain of terminal illness.

We will now define some of the terms that will be used in this session.

Analgesics – these are drugs used to relieve the symptoms of pain.

Non-steroidal anti-inflammatory drugs (NSAIDs) – this is the name given to a large number of different drugs which share certain pharmacological properties, such as interrupting the inflammatory response through one mechanism or another. Some drugs in this group also have analgesic properties and act to lower the body temperature in fever (for example, aspirin).

Opiate – a drug derived from the juice of the opium poppy, this includes morphine and codeine.

Opioid – a drug that acts as an opioid receptor and whose action is reversed by a morphine antagonist such as naloxone.

Opioid receptor – there are three main types: mu, delta and kappa. Each produces analgesia with a different spectrum of effects, including a variety of side effects.

Partial agonist/antagonist – a range of drugs which only partially inhibit or stimulate at the opioid receptor.

Opioid antagonist – a drug that reverses the effects of morphine and other agonists at the receptors.

2: Non-steroidal anti-inflammatory drugs (NSAIDs)

This is a diverse group of drugs that have different clinical structures but share similar therapeutic actions and side effects. This makes it convenient to treat them together. They have three main therapeutic actions.

● NSAIDs interrupt the inflammatory response by a number of different mechanisms: they are anti-inflammatory.

● Some NSAIDs lower body temperature in fever without affecting normal body temperature: they are antipyretic.

● Most NSAIDs are moderate modifiers of the pain response. Part of their action is a reduction of the levels of chemical mediators of inflammation that influence the nociceptors. They also have some action on the central nervous system – they are analgesics. Some, such as indomethacin, are relatively weak analgesics.

The prototype drug within this group is aspirin and all the chemical components which share the above pharmacological properties, irrespective of their chemical structure, were once referred to as aspirin-like drugs. These drugs are now more commonly known as non-steroidal anti-inflammatory drugs (NSAIDs). Examples of these drugs are aspirin, indomethacin, diflunisal, sulindac, diclofenac, ibuprofen and naproxen.

These drugs will normally have the following effects:

● they lower body temperature in fever, with no effect on normal body temperature

● they are powerful anti-inflammatory drugs in the treatment of conditions such as rheumatoid arthritis

● they are very good analgesics, but are better at relieving pain in headaches, bone pain and arthritis than visceral pain arising from the hollow organs of the body

● they are powerful inhibitors of blood platelet aggregation and are the first line of treatment for patients recovering from a heart attack and for prevention of a thrombosis in 'at risk' patients

● they may produce dose-related gastric ulceration and bleeding.

Mechanisms of action of this group of drugs

The majority of the therapeutic effects of these drugs, as well as most of their side effects, can be explained by their ability to inhibit the enzyme cyclo-oxygenase and so prevent the synthesis of prostaglandins. The prostaglandins are a family of biologically active fatty acids that act as important chemical mediators in a wide variety of physiological functions. However, they are also produced inappropriately or in excess during inflammation and tissue damage, becoming important mediators of the inflammatory responses and the development of nociceptive hypersensitivity.

We will now relate the mode of action of aspirin to its major pharmacological effects.

Lowering the body temperature in fever

During fever, a prostaglandin P.G.E.$_2$ is produced in the brain and causes the temperature regulatory centre in the hypothalamus to raise body temperature. Aspirin inhibits P.G.E.$_2$ production so that body temperature falls.

ACTIVITY 2 // ALLOW 5 MINUTES

In light of the information given so far in this session about aspirin, what do you think is the role of P.G.E.$_2$ in the control of normal body temperature?

Commentary

As aspirin does not lower normal body temperature but only lowers body temperature when it is elevated in fever, this suggests that P.G.E.$_2$ does not have any role in the control of normal body temperature.

Anti-inflammatory action

During inflammation, prostaglandins and other derivatives of arachidonic acid are produced and contribute to the pain, swelling and tissue damage. Aspirin inhibits their formation.

Analgesic action

The ability of aspirin to control pain occurs both through a peripheral and a central action. When aspirin inhibits the synthesis of prostaglandins in inflamed tissue it prevents the prostaglandins from sensitising the nociceptors. By inhibiting prostaglandin synthesis in the brain, aspirin is thought to also modify transmission in the pain conducting pathways.

Anti-platelet effect

The formation of the coronary thrombosis that leads to a heart attack is the result of the blood platelets sticking together to form a clot inside a blood vessel. Platelet aggregation is mediated by the prostaglandin thromboxane. Low doses of aspirin inhibit the platelet cyclo-oxygenase system, thereby suppressing the platelet clamping.

Gastric bleeding

Aspirin causes damage to the gastric mucosa partly by inhibiting the formulation of prostaglandins that protect the stomach wall from gastric acid.

Therapeutic uses of NSAIDs

NSAIDs are used clinically for:

● anti-inflammatory action in the treatment of muscle-skeletal conditions such as rheumatoid arthritis, osteoarthritis and so on

● their analgesic effects against pain of low to moderate intensity.

Aspirin and ibuprofen are available as over-the-counter drugs for a variety of aches and pains such as headaches, toothache and dysmenorrhoea.

Adverse reactions

All the NSAIDs share a common spectrum of adverse reactions. A number of these reactions are believed to be related to the inhibition of beneficial prostaglandin synthesis.

ACTIVITY 3 // **ALLOW 5 MINUTES**

From your experience, identify the possible short and long-term side effects for a patient taking NSAIDs.

Commentary

We discuss the possible side effects of NSAIDs below.

Gastrointestinal effects

The gastrointestinal side effects of NSAIDs occur most commonly in the stomach and include:

● dyspepsia or indigestion

● erosion of the mucosal membranes lining the stomach

● gastric ulcer formation

● perforation and haemorrhage of existing ulcers.

It has been estimated that in the USA there are over 2,500 deaths and 20,000 hospital admissions each year as the result of gastric side effects of NSAIDs in patients with rheumatoid arthritis. Similar studies in the UK have demonstrated that a significant minority of patients admitted with acute gastric pain had taken NSAIDs in the previous 24 hours.

The adverse effects of NSAIDs on the stomach are more marked in elderly females. This is because oestrogen and progesterone have beneficial effects on the gastric mucosa and these hormones are lost after the menopause. Thinning of the gastric mucosa occurs in both sexes with age and this probably results in the stomach becoming more susceptible to damage from the ingestion of NSAIDs.

Other side effects

NSAIDs produce a variety of renal effects, including decreased renal blood flow and glomerular filtration. For this reason NSAIDs are contra-indicated or used with caution in patients with impairment of renal function.

NSAIDs produce sodium retention, which is in part due to decreased glomerular filtration but is also due to inhibition of renal prostaglandin synthesis, which enhances the reabsorption of sodium.

NSAIDs also produce tinnitus (ringing in the ears) and impairment of hearing at high doses.

Drug interactions

NSAIDs are widely prescribed in the elderly for conditions such as arthritis. However, this group of patients is also likely to have multiple organ dysfunction and may therefore be taking a wide variety of other drugs. Although some particular NSAIDs have unique side effects and interaction with other drugs, there is a wide range of drug interactions that can occur with any NSAID.

- All NSAIDs decrease digoxin clearance by the kidney, thus increasing the risk of digoxin toxicity in patients with renal impairment.

- All NSAIDs decrease the renal clearance of lithium.

- All NSAIDs decrease the clearance of anti-neoplastic doses of methatrixate.

- Anion-exchange resins, such as cholestryamine used to lower blood cholesterol, bind NSAIDs in the intestine so reducing their therapeutic effectiveness in binding cholesterol.

- NSAIDs reduce the effect of antihypertensive drugs. This is probably due to their effect in causing sodium retention.

- NSAIDs are contra-indicated in patients being treated with oral anticoagulant therapy. This is because NSAIDs displace the anticoagulant drugs from their binding sites at the plasma proteins, leading to a massive increase in the plasma concentration of the unbound drugs. This leads to an increased risk of haemorrhage.

3: The use of NSAIDs in pain control

NSAIDs are weak analgesic drugs whose main action is to suppress inflammation and pain by blocking prostaglandin synthesis. They are particularly useful in blocking pain in situations in which injury or inflammation produce prostaglandins that sensitise nociceptors to normally painless mechanical or chemical stimuli.

Paracetamol

Paracetamol is not a non-steroidal anti-inflammatory drug. However, like NSAIDs it will reduce temperature in fever and is an effective analgesic. It does not have anti-inflammatory actions and only weakly inhibits cyclo-oxygenase. Like aspirin, paracetamol is a widely available analgesic but may be toxic, especially if used in higher than recommended doses. The number of suicides attributed to the drug has increased alarmingly in recent years and acute overdose may cause fatal liver damage at a dose level of l0 to l5 gr., which is two or three times the maximum dose of 4 gr. per day recommended for pain control.

ACTIVITY 4   // **ALLOW 10 MINUTES**

If you consider the range of side effects that may occur with NSAIDs, what would be some of the information you should obtain from a patient before starting treatment?

Commentary

Before treatment starts you should check for contra-indications such as:

- haemophilia
- gastrointestinal ulceration
- breastfeeding
- children under 12.

You should also undertake the following:

- assess the patient's vital signs, including heart rate and hearing
- assess for signs of gastrointestinal upsets or bleeding
- assess pain levels and the patient's experience of pain
- obtain a full record of the patient's medication, including self-medication.

ACTIVITY 5   // **ALLOW 10 MINUTES**

During treatment it is obviously good nursing practice to regularly evaluate a patient's responses to drugs in order to check the effectiveness of the therapy and the development of any adverse reactions. Make a note of some of the factors that you think are important to check in a patient being treated with relatively high doses of aspirin for rheumatism.

Commentary

The patient's response to the drug could be assessed by asking the patient about pain control and assessing whether the patient's mobility has improved since starting the treatment.

In relation to side effects it would be important to find out whether the patient had any gastric pain and to assess the possibility of fluid and salt retention by checking the patient's weight. It would also be important to ask the patient about hearing levels.

4: Opioid analgesics

The term 'opioid' is used to describe a group of drugs that are opium-like or morphine-like in their properties.

ACTIVITY 6	// ALLOW 15 MINUTES

Morphine-like drugs mimic the action of a group of natural substances found in the brain and other areas of the body. What are these natural substances?

Commentary

The natural substances which morphine-like drugs mimic are **enkephalins**, **endorphins** and **dynorphins** which act in the central nervous system to modify nociceptive pathways and reduce the sensation of pain.

Sources of opium

Historically the natural opioid drugs have been referred to as narcotic drugs, from the Greek word meaning stupor. This term was allied to a wide range of drugs, not just the opioids. With our increased understanding of the different activities of morphine the word narcotic is no longer used. The term 'opioid' is now used to describe all of these drugs.

Morphine is extracted from opium, which is the dried juice of the seed capsule of the opium poppy, papaver somniferum. Opium contains a large number of active drugs but therapeutic medical interest is primarily associated with two different classes of alkaloids present in the juice of the seed pod.

- The phenanthrene alkaloids, which include morphine and codeine. These alkaloids are strong analgesics and can produce sedation at high doses.

- The benzylisoquinoline alkaloids, of which papaverine is present in the highest concentration. These alkaloids are not analgesics but have a wide range of other pharmacological properties including vasodilation.

Synthetic opioid compounds

In addition to the natural alkaloids there is a large group of man-made opioid compounds used as analgesics. Although many of these were synthesised in an attempt to reduce the unwanted effects of morphine, such as tolerance and dependence, they share many of the properties of morphine. However, many of these compounds differ in their analgesic potency from morphine. These synthetic opioid drugs include diamorphine (heroin), methadone, pethidine, dihydrocodeine and dextropropoxphene (when combined with paracetamol this is known as co-proxamol).

Mechanism of action of opioids

Opioids exert their effects by binding with one or more opioid receptors. The most important receptors in producing the analgesic and other major effects of opioid drugs are the mu and kappa receptors.

Pharmacological properties of opioid-like drugs

Because all opioid drugs share a similar spectrum of pharmacological activity we will look at the pharmacology of morphine in detail as a representative drug for the whole group. We will then mention one or two of the other drugs to indicate where they differ significantly in their effects from morphine.

Morphine and related drugs produce analgesia predominantly by acting as agonists at the mu receptor, although they also interact powerfully with the kappa and delta receptors.

Effects of morphine on the central nervous system

Morphine has the following effects on the central nervous system.

- In patients with severe pain, morphine produces analgesia and increased tolerance to pain. At higher doses drowsiness, euphoria and mental clouding can occur. Other sensations such as touch are not affected. A number of patients can still locate the pain but the perception of pain and emotional stress associated with it are removed by the morphine.

- In the majority of pain-free individuals the over-administration of morphine can produce dysphoria, anxiety and vomiting.

- On first-dose administration, morphine stimulates the chemoreceptor trigger zone in the medulla oblongata to produce a feeling of nausea and even vomiting. In most patients this effect is not seen on subsequent administration.

- Morphine produces marked constriction of the pupil of the eye – miosis – through central nervous system stimulation. Pinpoint pupils can be taken as a diagnostic sign of over-dosage before respiratory depression becomes apparent.

- Morphine is a powerful respiratory depressant, particularly in neonates. It acts upon the respiratory centre in the medulla oblongata to reduce its responsiveness to carbon dioxide. Death from toxic overdose of morphine is normally the result of respiratory depression.

- Morphine is a potent cough suppressant through suppression of the cough reflex.

- Morphine has a biphasic effect on body temperature. Low doses can decrease body temperature, but high doses increase body temperature.

Effects on the gastrointestinal tract – long-term use

Long-term use of morphine has the following effects on the gastrointestinal tract:

- Morphine produces severe constipation by blocking intestinal propulsive peristalsis and decreasing gastric motility.

- The secretion of hydrochloric acid in the stomach and biliary, pancreatic and intestinal digestive system are decreased, delaying the digestion of food.

- Constriction of the sphincter of Oddi causes an increase in pressure in the bile duct. Patients with biliary colic may thus experience an increase rather than a decrease in pain when given morphine.

Effects on other smooth muscle

Use of morphine has the following effects on other smooth muscle.

- Morphine has a dual effect on the bladder. It increases detrusor muscle tone, producing a feeling of urinary urgency. However, at the same time it also increases sphincter tone, making voiding difficult. Tolerance to these effects of morphine on the bladder develops, but sometimes patients require catheterisation at the beginning of treatment.

- Morphine can prolong labour by affecting the uterus.

ACTIVITY 7   **// ALLOW 10 MINUTES**

Considering the wide-ranging effects that morphine has on the central nervous system, can you think of any problems that may arise if morphine is used as an analgesic during labour?

Commentary

Excluding the direct effect upon the uterine smooth muscle, morphine has two potential hazards, one on the mother and the other on the neonate.

- The central effects of morphine on the mother may reduce her will to cooperate in the delivery, so prolonging the labour and increasing risk of neonatal mortality.

- In the neonate there is great danger of fatal respiratory depression, since neonates are particularly sensitive to the respiratory depressive effects of morphine.

Histamine release by morphine

Morphine releases histamine from mast cells and other sites throughout the body and this has a number of effects which are mainly allergic reactions. In the bronchioles the release of histamine can cause broncho-constriction. This, combined with the respiratory depression produced by morphine, can make breathing difficult. In the skin, morphine can cause dilation of the surface blood vessels leading to flushing. Also, the release of histamine in the skin can give an itchy sensation that is most uncomfortable.

5: Therapeutic action of opioids

ACTIVITY 8 // **ALLOW 15 MINUTES**

As you have seen, opioids have widespread pharmacological actions. Taking these into consideration, list three major therapeutic uses for morphine or its derivatives.

Commentary

Three major therapeutic uses for opioids are as follows.

● **Analgesia**, particularly in severe acute and chronic pain: for example, in myocardial infarction, traumatic injury, surgery or terminal illness.

● **Controlling diarrhoea**: however, a drug such as loperamide, which acts locally in the intestine, may be preferred. (Loperamide is poorly absorbed so it produces constipation without analgesia, respiratory depression or drug dependency).

● **Cough suppression**: morphine and its derivatives are the most potent drugs known to suppress the cough centre in the medulla oblongata. It is also possible to separate the cough suppression activity of the opioid drugs from their analgesic action and potential to produce dependence. Codeine effectively suppresses cough at blood concentrations lower than those required to suppress pain. The synthetic drug dextromethophan suppresses cough but has no analgesic, respiratory depressant or central nervous system stimulating activity.

Adverse reactions

ACTIVITY 9 // ALLOW 15 MINUTES

From a consideration of the pharmacology of the opioids described above, suggest four or five of the most common side effects that can occur at therapeutic dose levels.

Commentary

Some of the most common side effects of opioids are as follows.

- **Constipation**. This occurs, to a greater or lesser extent, in most patients receiving these drugs. The use of regular prophylactic laxatives is therefore always indicated when opioids are administered.

- **Respiratory depression**. This is also common. It is dose-dependent and results from depression of the respiratory centre in the medulla oblongata.

- **Nausea** and **vomiting**. This particular response is common at the start of medication, but as treatment continues the patient rapidly becomes tolerant to this action of morphine.

- **Allergic reactions** due to the release of histamine.

- **Broncho-constriction** due to the release of histamine.

- Increase in **biliary pressure** leading to increased abdominal pain.

- Increased risk of **dependence** and **tolerance**. However, the risk of drug dependence is surprisingly low with the therapeutic use of opioids.

Morphine substitutes

Heroin (diamorphine)

Heroin is diacetylated morphine and is about three times as potent as morphine as an analgesic. It has a more rapid onset of analgesic action but a shorter duration of action. It is the drug of choice for subcutaneous administration due to its high water solubility. This permits the administration of high concentrations of the drug in a small injection volume. Heroin is a very powerful drug of dependence. Its manufacture, sale and use, even in clinical situations, are illegal in the USA. Heroin is normally used when morphine is ineffective in pain control.

Codeine

This has pharmacological effects similar to morphine, with about one tenth of its potency. It is also an excellent cough suppressant and produces less respiratory depression than morphine and has a lower abuse potential. Low dose preparations are available as over-the-counter medicines.

Pethidine

Although less potent than morphine, pethidine has a number of advantages. It has less effect than morphine on the cough or respiratory centres and is not constipating. It is preferred to morphine in labour where it is shorter acting and has less depressant effect on neonatal respiration.

Mixed agonist/antagonist opioids

These drugs were developed in an attempt to produce morphine-like analgesic drugs which do not produce euphoria and which are therefore less liable to abuse. In varying degrees they share all the pharmacological effects of morphine, such as analgesia, respiratory depression, cough suppression, nausea and vomiting.

Methadone

Methadone is more effective after oral administration than morphine and has a longer duration of action but about the same potency. The major difference between morphine and methadone is that methadone does not produce euphoria. It also suppresses the withdrawal symptoms characteristic of opioid drug dependence and blocks the euphoric effect of heroin and morphine. Both tolerance and physical dependence can occur with methadone as with most opioids, but these are less severe.

6: Tolerance, dependence and withdrawal symptoms

In pharmacological terms the three characteristics of tolerance, dependence and withdrawal symptoms are different aspects of drug action. However, because these characteristics are often linked together it is probably more convenient to deal with them together.

ACTIVITY 10   // ALLOW 10 MINUTES

Write down what you think is meant by the term 'tolerance to the pharmacological or therapeutic effects of a drug'.

Commentary

Tolerance to the pharmacological or therapeutic effects of a drug is a widespread phenomenon. It is seen in situations where increasing concentrations of the drug have to be given to maintain the same level of efficacy or effectiveness as originally seen with a lower dose. Most cases of tolerance arise due to faulty dose administration, which usually means that too much of the drug is being prescribed too frequently.

There are a number of different mechanisms by which the body can become tolerant to the actions of a drug. The two most common are as follows.

● Increased metabolism of the drug due to enzyme activity in the liver. This means that there is less drug available at its site of action and increased doses have to be given to maintain the same level of therapeutic effect. This type of tolerance is seen with the barbiturates.

● Time-related changes in receptor sensitivity. With the opioids, repeated high dose administration leads to tolerance of the analgesic, euphoric and respiratory depressant action of the drugs. There is partial tolerance to the constipating effects of the drug but tolerance does not develop to the papillary constriction.

Withdrawal symptoms

If opioids are suddenly withdrawn from a tolerant individual then within one or two hours the individual starts exhibiting withdrawal symptoms.

ACTIVITY 11 // **ALLOW 15 MINUTES**

The symptoms of withdrawal are generally the opposite to the physiological effects seen following the administration of morphine. Considering the major actions of morphine, list some of the symptoms you might expect to see in a patient exhibiting morphine withdrawal.

Commentary

Your list may include some or all of the following:

● dysphoria and increased sensitivity to pain and touch

● increase in secretions from nose, mouth and gastrointestinal tract

● diarrhoea and severe intestinal cramps

● widely dilated pupils

● respiratory and cardiovascular stimulation.

The severity of the withdrawal symptoms can be reduced or abolished by withdrawing the opioid slowly through gradually reducing the daily intake.

Dependence and substance abuse

Drug dependence is characterised by drug-seeking behaviour that takes precedence over other forms of behaviour. In its extreme form the entire existence of the individual concerned becomes tied up with drug-seeking behaviour. Drug dependence is most commonly associated with the development of tolerance and physical dependence. However, drug dependence is rarely seen in individuals receiving opioids for the therapeutic relief of pain, even though they exhibit tolerance to the drugs resulting from the administration of high doses.

7: Other drugs used in the treatment of pain

In palliative care a small number of drugs which are not classified either clinically or pharmacologically as analgesic drugs are used to relieve pain. Why such drugs should act as analgesics in some patients is unknown, and their use in palliative care often involves non-licensed indications, routes and dosages. Not all patients respond to these drugs and they are always introduced into treatment as an adjutant after treatment with powerful drugs such as morphine has failed to provide complete pain relief for the patient. When the decision has been made to use adjutant drugs, the starting dose should be low and the patient should be carefully monitored.

Anti-convulsants

Anti-convulsant drugs are useful in some types of neuropathic pain. There is no drug of choice but garbamazine and sodium valproate are commonly used. However, in the elderly, anti-convulsant drugs used in relatively high doses can produce sedation and dizziness.

Anti-depressants

Anti-depressant drugs such as imipramine have also proven useful as an adjutant in neuropathic pain. As with the anti-depressant action of these drugs, it takes seven to ten days after treatment before any therapeutic effect becomes noticeable. A mild but very uncomfortable side effect in terminal patients is a dry mouth.

Corticosteroids

Patients with bone pain can obtain additional pain relief by using steroids such as dexamethasone as an adjutant.

Before you move on to Session Nine, check that you have achieved the objectives given at the beginning of this session and, if not, review the appropriate sections.

The practice of pain management

Introduction

In this session we look at the management of pain. We start by considering the World Health Organisation analgesic ladder of pain management. We then look in more detail at the use of drugs in pain management and we consider drug dependence and 'the pain habit'.

Session objectives

When you have completed this session you should be able to:

● describe appropriate drug regimes for the relief of acute and chronic pain

● outline the characteristics of drug dependence in patients being treated with potent analgesics such as morphine

● explain the term 'the pain habit' and discuss how this situation can be prevented

● describe ways in which 'wind-up' can be avoided in surgical and terminal pain.

1: Relief of pain

The management of pain is one of the most important and, as we have seen, difficult issues in nursing practice. The purpose of drugs in pain control is to keep the patient completely free of pain and this is probably best achieved by applying the World Health Organisation analgesic ladder of pain management.

Step 1 – if the patient is not on analgesics then start with paracetamol, aspirin or a similar non-opioid analgesic.

Step 2 – if Step 1 drugs fail to control pain then give the patient weak opioid analgesics such as dihydrocodeine or co-proxamol.

Step 3 – if pain is not controlled by Step 2 drugs, then start the patient on potent opioid analgesics, such as morphine or diamorphine.

In many ways this strategy is more applicable to surgical and traumatic pain and should not be used unthinkingly in patients with unreasonable chronic pain: uncritical adherence to this, or any other general protocol may not assist the carer in deriving the best care for the individual patient. The strict application of the above treatment protocol would do little to provide relief to a patient in chronic pain with all the complications of spinal 'wind-up'.

2: Choice of drugs

The choice of drugs used to relieve pain is very wide. Obviously if we can identify the cause of the pain then the drug of choice is the drug that removes that particular cause.

ACTIVITY 1 // ALLOW 10 MINUTES

Identify drugs which are not analgesics, but which can bring about relief from pain by dealing with its causes.

Commentary

Examples of drugs which are not analgesics but which can relieve pain by dealing with its causes are:

- antacids used for the pain of heartburn or indigestion

- muscle relaxants which relieve muscle spasm associated with some painful conditions.

Unfortunately, most pain does not have such clearly defined causes and for the relief of the pain we have to administer drugs that act at various levels along the nociceptive pathways. This alleviates our subjective experience of the sensation of pain but not the cause of the pain itself.

Some examples of drug regimens

Acute short-term pain

This pain is almost always the result of accidental or surgical trauma. It normally starts off as fairly intense and decreases as the patient recovers.

ACTIVITY 2   **// ALLOW 10 MINUTES**

After surgery or acute accidental trauma, pain can sometimes be absent or much less than would be expected from the extent of the tissue damage. Can you suggest why this may occur?

Commentary

This may occur because:

- after surgery, the patient is still experiencing the residual effects of the anaesthetic drugs administered during surgery

- in acute trauma, the ascending pain pathways in the spinal cord are suppressed, resulting from the emotional stress of the accident.

In acute short-term pain, the patient's maximum experience of pain will occur two to three days after tissue damage when the inflammatory response is at its peak. A suitable dose regimen would therefore be to prescribe a strong opioid analgesic by injection, combined with an oral non-steroidal anti-inflammatory drug (NSAID) for the first week to relieve the acute severe pain. These drugs should be administered before the patient reports severe pain in order to inhibit development of 'wind-up' in the nociceptive pathways in the spinal cord. As the patient recovers, the strong opioids can be replaced by non-opioid analgesics.

Chronic pain

The patient's experience of chronic pain can vary widely, and in general the weakest possible drugs necessary to control the pain are used. If the severity of the pain increases then stronger drugs are employed, following the guidelines laid down in the analgesic ladder of pain management.

ACTIVITY 3   **// ALLOW 10 MINUTES**

Make a list of the pharmacological factors arising from the use of analgesic drugs which you think may complicate the management of pain.

Commentary

In chronic pain the patient will be receiving analgesic drugs continuously. This can give rise to a number of complications in the management of the patient and his or her pain. The following are common complications:

- development of drug tolerance

- development of drug dependence

- possibility of the development of side effects arising from long-term medication – for example, liver or kidney damage

- development of 'wind-up'.

You should now read *Resource 6* from the *Resources Section*, which explores one particular form of treatment for chronic pain at greater length.

3: Drug dependence

The social and psychological problems seen with street addicts of opioid analgesics are exceedingly rare in patients being treated with this class of drugs. However, the following characteristics of drug dependence can sometimes be observed.

- Physical dependence. This is characterised by tolerance to the drug and withdrawal symptoms when the drug is discontinued.

- Psychological dependence. This is characterised by a need for the drug to achieve emotional well-being. This most often arises due to the practice of under-medicating the patient, which leads to pain breakthrough. In this situation the patient only experiences pain relief after dose administration and this leads to 'craving' for the drug to bring about pain relief.

ACTIVITY 4   **// ALLOW 10 MINUTES**

Can you suggest ways in which nursing practice can reduce the incidence of drug dependence?

Commentary

The danger of both physical and psychological dependence in drug treatment can be reduced by titration (continuous measurement and adjustment) of the dose and time of administration to the patient's individual needs. This means that the patient is kept pain-free at the lowest possible concentration of the drug. It is also important that the patient is provided with an emotionally supportive nursing environment in order to assist in minimising the perception of pain.

4: The pain habit

This phrase normally refers to the patient's experience of incomplete pain relief when analgesic drugs are being administered according to a fixed dose schedule that does not properly consider the patient's individual needs. When a patient with severe pain does not receive sufficient analgesia to provide total relief then as the pain 'breaks through' the patient will begin to experience the initial stages of 'wind-up'. The patient will then start to make demands for stronger and more powerful analgesics, and want the dose more frequently. The patient can then be described as having a 'pain habit' resulting from the development of 'wind-up'.

ACTIVITY 5	// ALLOW 10 MINUTES

Recall some of the factors that contribute to the development of 'wind-up'.

Commentary

'Wind-up' refers to the increasing sensitivity of the nociceptive pathways to repetitive stimulation. It can occur through peripheral mechanisms at the level of the nociceptive receptor, or within the central nervous system or both.

Peripheral mechanism

This occurs when chemical mediators, such as histamine, prostaglandins and Substance P are released during inflammation or from damaged cells. These mediators combine with receptors that are close to the nociceptive nerve ending to lower their threshold to stimulation. The result is that the feeling of pain is increased as more impulses reach the central nervous system, and previously non-painful stimuli, such as touch, are now perceived as painful.

Central mechanism

In the spinal cord, and probably in other nociceptive pathways, the increase in impulse traffic through the synapses alters the normal synaptic transmission by causing the release of additional neurotransmitters. These neurotransmitters reduce the effectiveness of enkephalins in blocking the perception of pain, and so increase the patient's perception of the pain experience.

Unfortunately the conventional analgesic ladder of using the least potent drugs at the lowest possible dose is actually conducive to the development of 'wind-up'. Recent experience of treating terminally ill patients in hospice care suggests that an alternative approach may be more effective. In this, patients with chronic pain are treated aggressively with high doses of potent analgesics to achieve rapid and early control of pain. Once this is established and the patient is comfortable, then both the dose and type of analgesic employed are reduced in order to determine the minimum effective dose regimen needed to keep the patient pain-free.

Surgical pain

Clinical studies have demonstrated that giving morphine to women before rather than during or after surgery for hysterectomies reduces their post-operative need for analgesics by about a third. For further details of this you should read *Resource 7*. It also significantly reduced post-operative abdominal tenderness. This and other clinical trials indicate that giving morphine-like analgesics or local anaesthetics to block sensory input from a surgical wound site to the spinal cord is a more effective strategy than giving the drugs post-operatively when the patient is experiencing pain and spinal 'wind-up' has started.

Terminal pain

In many instances the principles adopted for the treatment of chronic pain also apply to terminal pain. Because a patient's life expectancy in these circumstances is limited, patient function, comfort and quality of life are primary considerations. Drugs of the required potency should be given before pain develops and the patient should be involved in these decisions for as long as possible. Regular dosing is essential and continuous analgesia by infusion provides very good pain control.

You should now check that you have achieved the objectives given at the beginning of this session and, if not, review the appropriate sections.

LEARNING REVIEW

You should use the list of learning outcomes given below to test the progress you have made in this unit. The list is an exact repeat of the one you completed at the beginning of the unit. You should tick the box on the scale that corresponds with the point you have reached now and then compare it with your scores on the learning profile you completed at the beginning of the unit. If there are any areas you are still unsure about you might like to review the sessions concerned.

	Not at all	Partly	Quite well	Very well

Session One

I can:

- describe a typical neurone ☐ ☐ ☐ ☐

- identify different types of neurone and explain their functions ☐ ☐ ☐ ☐

- explain the function of nerve endings ☐ ☐ ☐ ☐

- identify the electrical and chemical factors essential in the functioning of nerve tissue. ☐ ☐ ☐ ☐

Session Two

I can:

- summarise the functions of the central nervous system ☐ ☐ ☐ ☐

- identify the structure and function of the five main parts of the brain ☐ ☐ ☐ ☐

- explain the function of the ventricles of the brain ☐ ☐ ☐ ☐

- explain the role of the meninges and cerebrospinal fluid. ☐ ☐ ☐ ☐

	Not at all	Partly	Quite well	Very well

Session Three

I can:

- explain the structure and function of the spinal cord ❏ ❏ ❏ ❏

- identify the peripheral nerves ❏ ❏ ❏ ❏

- explain the type, function and distribution of the twelve cranial nerves ❏ ❏ ❏ ❏

- explain the function and route of the spinal nerves. ❏ ❏ ❏ ❏

Session Four

I can:

- explain the anatomical difference between a voluntary movement and a reflex action ❏ ❏ ❏ ❏

- explain the roles of the sympathetic and parasympathetic nervous systems ❏ ❏ ❏ ❏

- identify the functions of the autonomic nervous system. ❏ ❏ ❏ ❏

Session Five

I can:

- discuss the belief that pain is not a sensation but an emotion ❏ ❏ ❏ ❏

- identify the different types of pain and their physiological background ❏ ❏ ❏ ❏

- explain the functions of the two main types of nociceptor ❏ ❏ ❏ ❏

- discuss the value of superficial electrical stimulus in the control of acute pain ❏ ❏ ❏ ❏

- evaluate the stimulation of the brain and spinal cord in the control of pain. ❏ ❏ ❏ ❏

	Not at all	Partly	Quite well	Very well

Session Six

I can:

- describe the endogenous opioid system   ❏ ❏ ❏ ❏

- explain the role of the endogenous opioid system in the control of pain   ❏ ❏ ❏ ❏

- examine the role of acupuncture in pain control   ❏ ❏ ❏ ❏

- explain the pathophysiology of referred pain   ❏ ❏ ❏ ❏

- discuss the phenomenon of phantom or projected pain.   ❏ ❏ ❏ ❏

Session Seven

I can:

- distinguish between the three categories of pain   ❏ ❏ ❏ ❏

- explain the mechanisms which give rise to chronic pain   ❏ ❏ ❏ ❏

- discuss the concepts of hyperalgesia and secondary hyperalgesia   ❏ ❏ ❏ ❏

- discuss the notion of 'wind-up' as a major feature of chronic pain.   ❏ ❏ ❏ ❏

Session Eight

I can:

- identify the three main groups of analgesic drugs   ❏ ❏ ❏ ❏

- explain the main functions of non-opioid drugs   ❏ ❏ ❏ ❏

- explain the main mechanisms of the opioid drug groups   ❏ ❏ ❏ ❏

- discuss the use of adjutant drugs.   ❏ ❏ ❏ ❏

	Not at all	Partly	Quite well	Very well

Session Nine

I can:

- describe appropriate drug regimes for the relief of acute and chronic pain

| ❏ | ❏ | ❏ | ❏ |

- outline the characteristics of drug dependence in patients being treated with potent analgesics such as morphine

| ❏ | ❏ | ❏ | ❏ |

- explain the term 'the pain habit' and discuss how this situation can be prevented

| ❏ | ❏ | ❏ | ❏ |

- describe ways in which 'wind-up' can be avoided in surgical and terminal pain.

| ❏ | ❏ | ❏ | ❏ |

FURTHER READING

ANGELUCCI, D., QUINN, L. and HANDLIN, D. (1998) 'A pain management relief plan', *Nursing Management*, 29 (10): 45–54.

This article addresses a hospital's initiative to offer responsive pain management through the development of a pain management task force. It provides a sequential model and guide for nursing managers to use in their own healthcare environments.

BARBER, D. (1997) 'The physiology and pharmacology of pain: a review of opioids', *Journal of Perianaesthesia Nursing*, 12 (2): 95–99.

This article reviews the physiology of pain and the pharmacology of opioids.

BROCKOPP, D.Y., BROCKOPP, G., WARDEN, S., WILSON, J., CARPENTER, J.S. and VENDEVEER, B. (1998) 'Barriers to change: a pain management project', *International Journal of Nursing Studies*, 35 (4): 226–232.

This project was designed to examine barriers to the effective management of pain encountered in acute care settings. Results identified seven major barriers to pain management: lack of knowledge, non-facilitative attitudes, inconsistent leadership, poor working relationships, cultural and religious biases, physicians' fear of legal repercussions and a lack of resources.

CRAWLEY, I. and WEBSTER, C. (1998) 'Telephone help for chronic pain', *Practice Nurse*, 15 (5) 259–263.
    There never seems to be enough time in a GP or consultant appointment to discuss fears and concerns over pain and its management. The authors describe the work of the nurse-run pain helpline for patients with chronic non-terminal pain.

LIVNETH, J., GARBER, A. and SHAEVICH, E. (1998) 'Research study: assessment and documentation of pain in oncology patients', *International Journal of Palliative Nursing*, 4 (4): 169–175.

The study revealed that no procedures had been established to adequately deal with the management of pain and therefore the authors recommend that a pain assessment and documentation policy should be adopted in the care and treatment of all oncology patients.

McDONALD, D.D. and STERLING, R. (1998) 'Acute pain reduction strategies used by well older adults', *International Journal of Nursing Studies*, 35 (5): 265–270.

Thirty older adults, without chronic pain, were interviewed about the acute pain reduction strategies that they use at home and strategies that might be used if they were hospitalised. Results suggest that many older adults possess pain reduction strategies that may be helpful to incorporate in their pain management when hospitalised.

RICHARDS, S. (1997) 'Which analgesia? Guidelines to pharmacological pain control', *Professional Nurse*, 12 (9:sup.): 1–12.

The aim of this guide is to provide an accessible resource for nursing and medical staff on current pharmacological methods of pain control: the different types of analgesic that are available, the indications for each and their doses, formulations, contraindications and side effects.

WILKINSON, R. (1996) 'A non-pharmacological approach to pain relief', *Professional Nurse*, 11 (4): 222–224.

Effective pain management programmes must acknowledge the subjective nature of pain. Non-pharmacological pain management can be as effective, on occasions, as pharmacological pain management. Stress and anxiety evoke a similar physiological response to acute pain, highlighting the need for efficient cognitive management programmes.

TWYCROSS, A. (1988) 'The management of acute pain in children', *Professional Nurse*, 14 (2): 95–98.

Children cannot always articulate the level of pain they are experiencing, and need to be assessed carefully. This article discusses a number of pain assessment tools available to help nurses caring for children in pain.

USEFUL WEB
ADDRESSES
RELATED TO PAIN

A good starting point is the electronic journal, 'Online Pain', which can be found at **http://www.pain.com/onlinepainjournal/default.cfm**

Other useful sites include:

'Dee's pain management site' at **http://www.web-shack.com/dee/**

'RCN Pain Forum' at **http://www.jr2.ox.ac.uk:80/Bandolier/painres/painres.html**

'Worldwide Congress on Pain' at **http://www.pain.com/**

'COPE' (Center for Pain Education) at **http://members.tripod.com/~COPE_/**

'Adult Pain' site at **http://adultpain.nursing.uiowa.edu/**

The Yahoo directory lists a number of sites on the subject of chronic pain. These can be found at **http://www.yahoo.co.uk/Health/Diseases_and_Conditions/Chronic_Pain/**

RESOURCES SECTION

Contents page

Resource 1

Making Connections – The Synapse

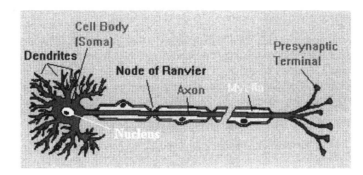

Neurons have specialized projections called dendrites and axons. Dendrites bring information to the cell body and axons take information away from the cell body.

Information from one neuron flows to another neuron across a synapse. The synapse is a small gap separating 2 neurons. The synapse consists of:

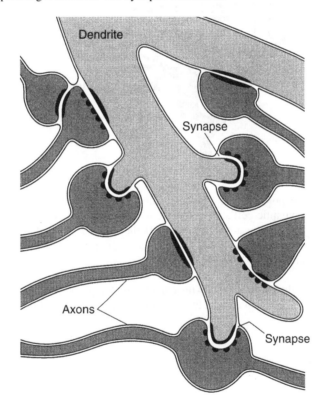

1. a presynaptic ending that contains neurotransmitters, mitochondria and other cell organelles,
2. a postsynaptic ending that contains receptor sites for neurotransmitters and,
3. the synaptic cleft: a space between the presynaptic and postsynaptic endings.

Electrical Trigger for Neurotransmission

For communication between neurons to occur, an electrical impulse must first travel down an axon to the synaptic terminal.

Neurotransmitter Mobilization and Release

Here at the synaptic terminal (the presynaptic ending), the electrical impulse will trigger the migration of vesicles (the red dots in the figure to the left) containing neurotransmitters toward the presynaptic membrane. The vesicle membrane will fuse with the presynaptic membrane releasing the neurotransmitters into the synaptic cleft. Until recently, it was thought that a neuron produced and released only one type of neurotransmitter. This was called "Dale's Law". However, there is now evidence that neurons can contain and release more than one kind of neurotransmitter.

Diffusion of Neurotransmitters Across the Synaptic Cleft

The neurotransmitter molecules then diffuse across the synaptic cleft where they can bind with receptor sites on the postsynaptic ending to influence the electrical response in the postsynaptic neuron. In the figure on the right, the postsynaptic ending is a dendrite (axodendritic synapse), but synapses can occur on axons (axoaxonic synapse) and cell bodies (axosomatic synapse).

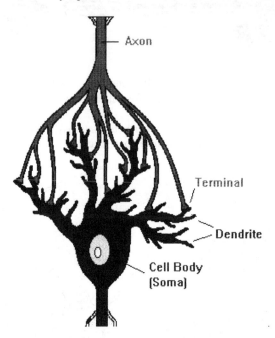

The response of the postsynaptic ending to the neurotransmitter binding results in a change in the postsynaptic cell's excitability: it will make the postsynaptic cell either more or less likely to fire an action potential. If the number of excitatory postsynaptic events are high enough, they will add to cause an action potential in the postsynaptic cell and a continuation of the "message".

Many psychoactive drugs and neurotoxins can change the properties of neurotransmitter release, neurotransmitter reuptake and the availability of receptor binding sites.

Resource 2

Action Potential

Neurons send messages through an electrochemical process. This means that chemicals result in an electrical signal. Chemicals in the body are "electrically-charged" - when they have an electrical charge, they are called "ions". The important ions in the nervous system are sodium and potassium (both have 1 positive charge, +), calcium (has 2 positive charges, ++) and chloride (has a negative charge, -). There are also some negatively charged protein molecules. It is also important to remember that nerve cells are surrounded by a membrane that allows some ions to pass through while it blocks the passage of other ions. This type of membrane is called semi-permeable.

Resting Membrane Potential

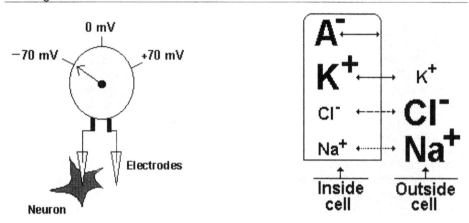

When a neuron is not sending a signal, it is said to be "at rest". When a neuron is at rest, the inside of the neuron is negative relative to the outside. While the concentrations of the different ions attempt to balance out on both sides of the membrane, they cannot because the cell membrane allows only some ions to pass through channels (ion channels). At rest, potassium ions (K+) can cross through the membrane easily. Also at rest, chloride ions (Cl-)and sodium ions (Na+) have a more difficult time crossing. The negatively charged protein molecules (A-) inside the neuron cannot cross the membrane. In addition to these selective ion channels, there is a pump that uses energy to move 3 sodium ions out of the neuron for every 2 potassium ions it puts in. Finally, when all these forces balance out, and the difference in the voltage between the inside and outside of the neuron is measured, you have the resting potential. The resting membrane potential of a neuron is about -70 mV (mV=millivolt) – this means that the inside of the neuron is 70 mV less than the outside. At rest, there are relatively more sodium ions outside the neuron and more potassium ions inside that neuron.

Action Potential

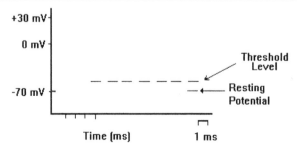

So the resting potential indicates what is happening with the neuron at rest. The action potential indicates what happens when the neuron transmits information from one cell to another. Neuroscientists use other words, such as a "spike" or an "impulse" to describe the action potential. The action potential is an explosion of electrical activity that is created by a depolarizing current. This means that some event (a stimulus) causes the resting potential to move toward 0 mV. When the depolarization reaches about -55 mV a neuron will fire an action potential. This is the threshold. If the neuron does not reach this critical threshold level, then no action potential will fire. Also, when the threshold level is reached, an action potential of a fixed sized will always fire...for any given neuron, the size of the action potential is always the same. There are no big or small action potentials in one nerve cell - all action potentials are the same size. Therefore, the neuron either does not reach the threshold or a complete action potential is fired - this is the "ALL OR NONE" principle.

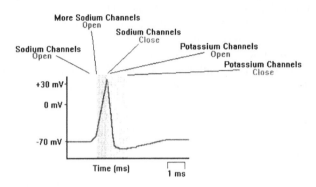

The "cause" of the action potential is an exchange of ions across the neuron membrane. A stimulus first results in the opening of sodium channels. Since there are a lot more sodium ions on the outside, and the inside of the neuron is negative relative to the outside, sodium ions rush into the neuron. Remember, sodium has a positive charge, so the neuron becomes more positive and becomes depolarized. It takes longer for potassium channels to open. When they do open, potassium rushes out of the cell, reversing the depolarization. Also at about this time, sodium channels start to close. This causes the action potential to go back toward -70 mV (a repolarization). The action potential actually goes past -70 mV (a hyperpolarization) since the potassium channels stay open a bit too long. Gradually, the ion concentrations go back to resting levels and the cell returns to -70 mV.

And there you have it...the Action Potential.

Management of the individual with pain

Gate Control Theory

In 1965, Melzack and Wall proposed that sensory perception is the result of activation of transmission (T) cells in the dorsal horn of the spinal cord, which in turn results from a balance of peripheral input along large-diameter (A-alpha and A-beta) and small-diameter (A-delta and C) afferent nerve fibers (Fig. 1). Activity from both large and small afferent neurons directly activates the T cell. However, noxious input transmitted via small-diameter fibers also inhibits inhibitory interneurons in the dorsal horn, thus decreasing the effect of presynaptic inhibition on the T cell from the interneurons and ultimately resulting in a net increase in perception of painful input.

In contrast, activity traveling along large-diameter afferent fibers activates the inhibitory interneurons, thus facilitating presynaptic inhibition of the T cell and ultimately resulting in a "closing of the spinal gate," or a decrease in the perception of sensory activity. In the early 1970s, transcutaneous electrical nerve stimulation (TENS) was viewed as a form of comfortable peripheral sensory input that could decrease pain perception by preferentially increasing the large-diameter afferent fiber input and facilitating presynaptic inhibition of the T cell, thus decreasing conscious pain perception. For instance, TENS has been demonstrated to be effective in relieving pain associated with postherpetic neuralgia, a disease that results in degeneration of large-diameter afferent fibers. Conventional TENS, when applied to the painful region or to a segmentally related region in which the population of large-diameter fibers remains intact, effectively controls the pain associated with postherpetic neuralgia by activating the remaining large-diameter afferent fibers that lie in close proximity to the pathologically active small-diameter afferent neurons in the neuraxis. Other analgesic treatment interventions, including massage or vibration, may also be explained by this theory.

The gate control theory was criticized for failing to 1) account for a variety of painful conditions in which small-diameter afferents were preferentially destroyed and 2) consider the role of higher centers in conscious pain perception. In 1968, Melzack and Casey suggested a modification of the gate control theory to account for activation of higher centers. They added the limbic and reticular systems, both of which are known to affect pain perception, emotional phases of affect, and motor responses. Higher centers in the neocortex also monitor painful afferent input by "comparing" it with past experiences and learned responses. Melzack and Casey suggested that a "central control trigger" activated by input to these higher centers might influence activity in the dorsal horn via descending systems and also might contribute to pain modulation. Thus, a mechanism for pain control via distraction, meditation, or relaxation was elucidated.

Stimulation-Produced Analgesia

A more recent theory of pain modulation is that of stimulation-produced analgesia (SPA), which involves the production and utilization of endogenous opiates, such as endorphins and enkephalins. In 1978, Basbaum and Fields proposed a negative feedback loop mechanism to account for analgesia resulting from low-frequency, high-intensity (acupuncture-like) TENS. They suggested that the noxious input associated with acupuncture-like TENS activates ascending pathways, leading to awareness of pain. Along these pathways, certain axons synapse within medullary reticular formation nuclei. Input from these nuclei then is transmitted to the periaqueductal gray (PAG) regions of the midbrain and thalamus, regions that have high concentrations of endogenous opiates and opiate receptors. When these regions are activated, efferent axons synapse within nuclei in the raphe magnus and reticularis gigantocellularis (RCG). Output from these nuclei descends in the spinal cord and makes enkephalinergic synapses that inhibit spinal transmission of Substance P, which is implicated as a neurotransmitter between axons conveying noxious information. Thus, the application of acupuncture-like TENS may activate a negative feedback loop that ultimately blocks further transmission of noxious information.

Because activation of endorphin-mediated analgesia may be blocked by naloxone, an opiate antagonist, analgesic procedures that are suspected of being endorphin mediated can be identified. Administration of naloxone will reverse this analgesia or return an elevated pain threshold to pretreatment values. Use of low-frequency, high-intensity electrical stimulation of acupuncture points and remote anatomical sites as an endorphin-mediated analgesia has been confirmed by some investigators and denied by others.

Analgesia resulting from acupuncture, acupressure, or cognitive interventions (eg, distraction, imagery, hypnosis) has also been associated with an endorphin-mediated mechanism. As methods of histochemical and electrophysiological data acquisition become more sophisticated, additional neurophysiological mechanisms (as well as confirmation or refutation of current ones) will add to our understanding of pain perception and modulation.

Motivational and Affective Components

Motivational and affective components influence an individual's perception of and response to pain. Factors that influence a person's emotional interpretation of and response to pain include age, sex, ethnicity, culture, religious background, attention and distraction levels, environment (eg, who's watching), and the response of others to his or her behavior. In addition, behavioral responses to pain depend on previous experience with pain, responses learned from others, and perception of control over the cause of the pain.

Acute vs Chronic Pain

Acute pain is often described as pain of less than 6 months duration for which an underlying pathology can be identified. Tissue inflammation, damage, or destruction is often related somatically, or in a referred distribution, to the location and intensity of the person's pain report. The pain is well localized and defined by the patient. Medication intake and other medical interventions usually are appropriate for the degree of pathology identified.

Acute pain is mediated through pathways that include rapidly conducting systems, such as the dorsal column postsynaptic system, spinocervical tract, and neospinothalamic tract. Acute pain is also associated with increases in muscle tone, heart rate, blood pressure, skin conductance, and other manifestations of increased sympathetic nervous system activity. In contrast, chronic pain appears to be mediated through slowly conducting fibers in the paleospinothalamic tract and spinoreticular formation and is often associated with insomnia, loss of appetite and libido, and feelings of helplessness and hopelessness, rather than with increased sympathetic nervous system activity.

Chronic pain is often of longer than 6 months duration. An underlying pathology is no longer identifiable and may never have been present. The patient's description of pain is less well defined and poorly localized, and objective physical findings are not identified. The patient's verbal description of the pain may contain words associated with emotional or motivational characteristics, in contrast to the predominance of sensory descriptors associated with acute pain. The patient may exemplify suffering through facial grimacing, stooped posture, antalgic gait, and verbal complaints that are out of proportion to the degree of pathology that may be identified. Self-imposed limited activity a disrupted lifestyle and avoidance of work, interaction with others, and sexual activity often is evident. Secondary gains such as monetary benefit, sympathy and attention from significant others, or avoidance of undesirable employment are present. Progressive inactivity, depression, anxiety, prescription drug misuse, and increased dependence on the health care system are all associated with the chronic pain experience.

Bond described physical pain as having characteristics analogous to those of acute pain. He labeled the poorly defined chronic pain experience as psychogenic pain, emphasizing that physical pain is usually alleviated once the underlying pathology has been identified and treated, whereas psychogenic pain is often unresponsive to physiological interventions.

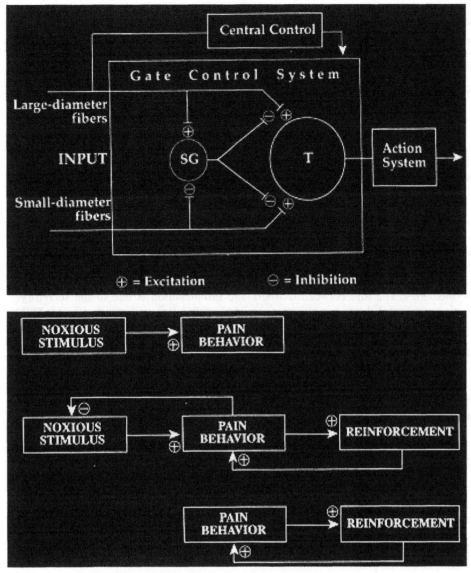

Figure 1: The gate control theory of pain modulation.

Resource 4

Pain Digest, 4(2):100-105, 1994. 69 References Service Anesthesiologie, IMC
Ixelles-Etterbeck, Brussels, Belgium (Dr M Sosnowski) GM.01 DC9416/346
© 1994

Pathophysiology of acute pain

In the normal human being, the identification of a sensation as being painful is a
function of higher associative centers in the brain in response to afferent impulses from
the periphery. The term "nociception" is used to describe the neural response to stimuli
potentially damaging to the individual. Before these afferents reach the brain and are
recognized as painful, a considerable amount of processing has already taken place,
both in the periphery and spinal cord.

Knowledge of the mechanisms of activation of nociceptors remains limited. Mechanical
and thermal receptors are probably activated directly by the stimulus. The activation of
polymodal nociceptors is potentiated by a variety of substances that may act as
intermediaries. The link between C fibers and inflammation is due to the secretory
functions of these fibers, not always associated with reflex or sensory effects. This
"axon flare" can equally be evoked by antidromic stimulation intense enough to activate
C fibers and is prevented by pretreatment with capsaicin, a neurotoxin that is selective
for neuropeptide-containing small-diameter fibers. The substance most prevalent in
vesicles isolated from terminals of small-diameter fibers, both centrally and
peripherally, is the neuropeptide substance P. The effect of the release of
proinflammatory agents is to sensitize adjacent nociceptors, resulting in an increase in
the spontaneous activity of some nociceptors that can produce membrane depolarization
of dorsal horn neurons. This cascade of peripheral changes in sensitivity is too small to
account for all the injury-induced alterations. It appears the inflammation process,
together with an increase in afferent barrage, initiates some central changes.

It has been shown that local application of lidocaine will stop the development of
secondary hyperalgesia. The analgesic actions of anti-inflammatory agents may provide
a new approach to the production of new analgesic drugs. The presence of opioid and a2
receptors on the terminals of unmyelinated nerves also is of therapeutic importance. The
role of adrenergic receptors on peripheral nociceptors probably plays a role in states of
enduring or chronic pain.

Pain from muscles and joints is evoked by a variety of stimuli including mechanical,
thermal, or chemical stimuli. Visceral pain is evoked by smooth muscle spasm,
ischemia, inflammation, and other chemical stimuli as well as mechanical stimuli.
Visceral nociceptive fibers run in sympathetic and parasympathetic nerves, and the pain
evoked by the activation of these fibers often has no precise localization. Not all viscera
contain specific nociceptors (brain), and it is not clear why specific nociceptors are
present in certain organs.

Recent evidence suggests that, in addition to the effects of tissue injury or noxious
stimulation on primary afferent neurons, there are also effects within the central nervous
system. Sensitization of dorsal horn neurons occurs after tissue injury or stimulation of
C-fiber afferent nerves with increasing frequency of neuronal activity in response to
repeated applications of the same noxious stimulus.

A noxious stimulus may also induce a hyperexcitable state of these neurons: a
progressive increase in dorsal-horn neuron response to repeated C-fiber stimulation
resulting in a prolonged discharge or "wind-up" of the cell. Brief afferent-conditioning
stimuli have recently been shown to induce prolonged changes in the receptive fields'
properties of dorsal horn neurons. In the spinal cord, hyperalgesia is produced by high-
frequency, C-fiber-strength electrical stimulation. In contrast, low-frequency or A-fiber-
strength stimulation will not produce hyperalgesia. This proposal is suggested by the C-
fiber neuropeptides being involved in triggering central sensitization and the evidence
implicating a contribution of excitatory amino acids to central sensitization. In addition,
an interaction of neuropeptides and excitatory amino acids is suggested by the finding
that intrathecal administration of substance P enhances the release of substances which

potentiate the effect of substance P. The author provides an in-depth description of the complex physiological process of hyperalgesia.

In addition to its role in enhancing pain transmission to central structures, the sensitization of spinal dorsal horn neurons also leads to an enhancement of spinal reflexes, including the flexion reflex. In summary, tissue injury sensitizes peripheral nociceptors, resulting in primary hyperalgesia. The release of neuropeptides such as substance P from the peripheral terminals of primary afferent C fibers leads to a spreading of inflammation and secondary hyperalgesia to uninjured tissue. One interesting suggestion was the role of nitric oxide in central sensitization. Nitric oxide may represent a new class of neurotransmitters, and drugs that interfere with its production may act as a new class of analgesics.

Resource 5

by Jeffrey A. Singer

Acupuncture, A Brief Introduction

In this paper I will be dealing with the ancient medical art of Acupuncture. Today in most western cultures it is considered a "new alternative" medicine. In reality Acupuncture (and its related Moxibustion) are practiced medical treatments that are over 5,000 years old. Very basically, Acupuncture is the insertion of very fine needles, (sometimes in conjunction with electrical stimulus), on the body's surface, in order to influence physiological functioning of the body.

Acupuncture can also be used in conjunction with heat produced by burning specific herbs, this is called Moxibustion. In addition, a non-invasive method of massage therapy, called Acupressure, can also be effective.

The first record of Acupuncture is found in the 4,700 year old Huang Di Nei Jing (Yellow Emperor's Classic of Internal Medicine). This is said to be the oldest medical textbook in the world. It is said to have been written down from even earlier theories by Shen Nung, the father of Chinese Medicine. Shen Nung documented theories about circulation, pulse, and the heart over 4,000 years before European medicine had any concept about them.

As the basis of Acupuncture, Shen Nung theorized that the body had an energy force running throughout it. This energy force is known as Qi (roughly pronounced Chee). The Qi consists of all essential life activities which include the spiritual, emotional, mental and the physical aspects of life. A person's health is influenced by the flow of Qi in the body, in combination with the universal forces of Yin and Yang . (I will discuss Yin and Yang a little later). If the flow of Qi is insufficient, unbalanced or interrupted, Yin and Yang become unbalanced, and illness may occur. Qi travels throughout the body along "Meridians" or special pathways. The Meridians, (or Channels), are the same on both sides of the body (paired). There are fourteen main meridians running vertically up and down the surface of the body. Out of these, there are twelve organ Meridians in each half of the body (remember they are in pairs). There are also two unpaired midline Meridians. There will be a diagram of Acupuncture points for treating diseases of the Meridians at the end of the digestive system paper. (See Appendix 1). The acupuncture points are specific locations where the Meridians come to the surface of the skin, and are easily accessible by "needling," Moxibustion, and Acupressure. The connections between them ensure that there is an even circulation of Qi, a balance between Yin and Yang.

Energy constantly flows up and down these pathways. When pathways become obstructed, deficient, excessive, or just unbalanced, Yin and Yang are said to be thrown out of balance. This causes illness. Acupuncture is said to restore the balance.

Yin and Yang is an important theory in the discussion of Acupuncture treatment, in relation to the Chinese theory of body systems. As stated earlier Qi is an energy force that runs throughout the body. In addition, Qi is also prevalent throughout nature as well. Qi is comprised of two parts, Yin and Yang. Yin and Yang are opposite forces, that when balanced, work together. Any upset in the balance will result in natural calamities, in nature; and disease in humans. Yin is signified by female attributes, passive, dark, cold, moist, that which moves medially, and deficient of Yang. Yang is signified by male attributes, light, active, warm, dry, that which moves laterally, and deficient of Yin. Nothing is completely Yin or Yang. The most striking example of this is man himself. A man is the combination of his mother (Yin) and and his father (Yang). He contains qualities of both: This is the universal symbol describing the constant flow of yin and yang forces. You'll notice that within yin, there is Yang, and within Yang, there is the genesis of Yin. Whether or not you believe in Taoist philosophy, (which all this is based on), one thing is indisputable: Acupuncture works.

Acupuncturists can use as many as nine types of Acupuncture needles, though only six are commonly used today. These needles vary in length, width of shaft, and shape of head. Today, most needles are disposible. They are used once and disgarded in accordance with medical biohazard regulations and guidlines. There are a few different precise methods by which Acupuncturists insert needles. Points can be needled anywhere in the range of 15 degrees to 90 degrees relative to the skin surface, depending on the treatment called for. In most cases, a sensation, felt by the patient, is desired. This sensation, which is not pain, is called deqi (pronounced dah-chee). The following techniques are some which may be used by an Acupuncturist immediately following insertion: Raising and Thrusting, Twirling or Rotation, Combination of Raising/Thrusting and Rotation, Plucking, Scraping (vibrations sent through the needle), and Trembling (another vibration technique). Once again, techniques are carefully chosen based on the ailment.

There are a few related procedures that fall into the range of Acupuncture treatments. The first is Electro-Acupuncture. This is the using of very small electrical impulses through the Acupuncture needles. This method is generally used for analgesia (pain relief or prevention). The amount of power used is only a few micro amperes, but the frequency of the current can vary from 5 to 2,000 Hz. The higher frequencies are generally used for surgery (usually abdominal), and the lower frequencies for general pain relief. The first reported successful use of Electro-Acupuncture was in 1958 in China for a tonsillectomy. Today, it is a common method of surgical analgesia used in China. Other methods for stimulating Acupuncture points have used Lasers and sound waves (Sonopuncture). A very commonly used treatment in the United States is Auriculotherapy or Ear Acupuncture. The theory is that since the ear has a rich nerve and blood supply, it would have connections all over the body. For this reason, the ear has many Acupuncture points which correspond to many parts and organs of the body. Auricular Acupuncture has been successful in treating problems ranging from obesity to alcoholism, to drug addiction. There are numerous studies either completed, or currently going on which affirms Auricular Acupuncture's effectiveness. (These will be mentioned in detail later on in the paper.)

Another popular treatment method is Moxibustion, which is the treatment of diseases by applying heat to Acupuncture points. Acupuncture and Moxibustion are considered complimentary forms of treatment, and are commonly used together. Moxibustion is used for ailments such as bronchial asthma, bronchitis, certain types of paralysis, and arthritic disorders.

Cupping is another type of treatment. This is a method of stimulating Acupuncture points by applying suction through a metal, wood or glass jar, in which a partial vacuum has been created. This technique produces blood congestion at the site, and therefore stimulates it. Cupping is used for low backache, sprains, soft tissue injuries, and helping relieve fluid from the lungs in chronic bronchitis.

One of the most popular alternatives to Acupuncture is Acupressure. This is simply Acupuncture without needles. Stimulation of the Acupuncture points is performed with the fingers or an instrument with a hard ball shaped head. Another variation of Acupressure is Reflexology (also called Zone Therapy). This is where the soles of the feet and the posterio-inferior regions of the ankle joints are stimulated. Many diseases of the internal organs can be treated in this manner.

The question arises, how does Acupuncture work? Scientists have no real answer to this; as you know many of the workings of the body are still a mystery. There are a few prevailing theories.

1. By some unknown process, Acupuncture raises levels of triglycerides, specific hormones, prostaglandins, white blood counts, gamma globulins, opsonins, and overall anti-body levels. This is called the "Augmentation of Immunity" Theory.
2. The "Endorphin" Theory states that Acupuncture stimulates the secretions of endorphins in the body (specifically Enkaphalins).
3. The "Neurotransmitter" Theory states that certain neurotransmitter levels (such as Seratonin and Noradrenaline) are affected by Acupuncture.
4. "Circulatory" Theory: this states that Acupuncture has the effect of constricting or dilating blood vessels. This may be caused by the body's release of Vasodilaters (such as Histamine), in response to Acupuncture.

5. One of the most popular theories is the "Gate Control" Theory. According to this theory, the perception of pain is controlled by a part of the nervous system which regulates the impulse, which will later be interpreted as pain. This part of the nervous system is called the "Gate." If the gate is hit with too many impulses, it becomes overwhelmed, and it closes. This prevents some of the impulses from getting through. The first gates to close would be the ones that are the smallest. The nerve fibers that carry the impulses of pain are rather small nerve fibers called "C" fibers. These are the gates that close during Acupuncture.

In the related "Motor Gate" Theory, some forms of paralysis can be overcome by Acupuncture. This is done by reopening a "stuck" gate, which is connected to an Anterior Horn cell. The gate, when closed by a disease, stops motor impulses from reaching muscles. This theory was first stated by Professor Jayasuriya in 1977. In it he goes on to say:

"...one of the factors contributing to motor recovery is almost certainly the activation of spindle cells. They are stimulated by Gamma motor neurons. If Acupuncture stimulates the Gamma motor neurons, the discharge causes the contraction of Intrafusal Muscle fibers. This activates the Spindle cells, in the same way as muscle stretching. This will bring about muscle contraction."

There are many diseases that can be treated successfully by Acupuncture or its related treatments. The most common ailments currently being treated are: lower backache, Cervical Spondylosis, Condylitis, Arthritic Conditions, Headaches of all kinds (including migraine), Allergic Reactions, general and specific use for Analgesia (including surgery), and relief of muscles spasms. There have also been clinical trials in the use of Acupuncture in treating anxiety disorders and depression. Likewise, very high success rates have been found in treating addictions to alcohol, tobacco (nicotine) and "hard' drugs. Acupuncture can rid the body of the physical dependency, but can not rid the mind of the habit (psychological dependency). For this reason, Acupuncture treatment of addictions has not been fully successful.

Case Studies

Obviously, especially for a paper such as this, my research would not be complete without backing it up with some case studies. Here they are.

The National Institute on Drug Abuse (NIDA) has sponsored three studies examining the effectiveness of Acupuncture for the treatment of substance abuse.

The first was at the Lincoln Medical Medical Center in Bronx, NYC, New York. It was headed by Dr. Douglas Lipton, and completed in 1991. This study used Auricular Acupuncture on Crack Cocaine users. The study was split into groups, one getting the correct Acupuncture treatments, the other getting "placebo" Acupuncture (needles placed in the "wrong" spots). Urinalysis results showed that the subjects receiving the correct treatments had lowered their use of the drug, in as little as two weeks. This was verified by testing for cocaine metabolite levels. However, the reduction was not as significant as had been anticipated. *Note that no other type of treatment, such as counseling as given.

In two other studies currently going on, (the first by Dr. Janet Konefal of Miami School of Medicine; and the other by Dr. Milton Bullock at the Hennepin County Medical Center in Minneapolis), counseling combined with acupuncture is being tested. The preliminary results have been quite promising.

Additional studies, too numerous to mention here have proven the effectiveness of Acupuncture therapy in Nicotine addiction, (look in Bibliography for some case citings).

Between 1971 and and 1972 a series of doctors (Frank Z. Warren: New York University Medical Center; Pang L. Man and Calvin H. Chen: Northville State Hospital, Northville, Michigan), conducted seven surgeries at both Northville State Hospital and at Albert Einstein Medical Center. they used both standard Acupuncture and Electro-Acupuncture techniques. They found that in all cases of surgery (six invasive and one dental) these Acupuncture treatments were successful in stopping the pain of surgery without additional anesthetics. In only one case (a repair of an inguinal hernia) did the patient complain of "discomfort;" and only in one additional case did a patient (the same one) complain of post-operative pain.

In conclusion, I feel that Acupuncture should be considered a valid form of treatment alongside, not only other "alternative" forms of treatment, but also along side mainstream medicine. More and more insurance companies are discovering the cost effectiveness of Acupuncture. Unfortunately, many insurance companies still do not cover Acupuncture therapy, with the exception of Drug Addiction treatments; and then only if other therapies have been unsuccessful, or as part of another program. Part of the reason for this is that as of the writing of this paper, the Food and drug Administration classifies Acupuncture needles as "investigational" devices. However, since this paper was written, the FDA has reclassified acupuncture needles and so, now, one great block to insurance coverage has been removed.

Acupuncture Doctors are licensed independently in most states while some states require you to be a Medical Doctor to practice Acupuncture.

Acupuncture schools are federally accredited by the ACAOM (Accreditation Commission for Acupuncture and Oriental Medicine). This accreditation allows the school to offer federal guaranteed student loans.

Bibliography

Baxi, Dr. Nilesh and Dr.CH Asrani. *Speaking of: Alternative Medicine: Acupuncture.* New Dehli, India: Sterling Publishers Private Ltd, 1986.

Duke, Marc. *Acupuncture.* New York: Pyramid House Books, 1972.

Holden, Constance. "Acupuncture: Stuck on the Fringe." *Science*, May 6, 1994, pg 770.

Lever, Dr. Ruth. *Acupuncture For Everyone.* Middlesex, England: Penguin Books, Ltd, 1987.

Lipner, Maxine. "Different Strokes." *Women's Sports and Fitness*, May/June, 1993, pg 31, 32, 85.

Moss, Dr. Louis. *Acupuncture And You: A New Approach To Treatment Based On The Ancient Method of Healing.* London, England: Elek Publishers, 1972.

Nightingale, Michael. *The Healing Power of Acupuncture.* New York: Sterling Publishing Co. Inc, 1986.

Ponce, Pedro E. "Eastern Medicine Collides with Western Regulations at Mass. Acupuncture School." *The Chronicle of Higher Education*, October 27, 1993, pg A32.

Saslow, Linda. "Scores of Students Take Up Acupuncture at Center in Syosset." *New York Times*, November 6, 1994.

Warren, Dr. Frank Z. *Handbook of Medical Acupncture.* New York: Van Nostrand Reinhold Co., 1976.

Case Studies

Dr. Douglas Lipton:"Lincoln Clinic Study"; Dr. Janet Konefal:"Miami Study"; Dr. Milton Bullock: "Hennepin County Study." *U.S. Department of Health & Human Services, National Institutes of Health, Office of Human Services*, AM, Volume 1, Number 3, January, 1994.

Brewington, Vincent, et al. "Acupuncture as a Detoxification Treatment: An Analysis of Controlled Research." *Journal of Substance Abuse Treatment*, Volume 11, Number 4, 1994, pg 289-307.

Professor Jayasuriya: Paper for the 5th World Congress of Acupuncture;1977: Tokyo, Japan

Resource 6

Antidepressants and chronic pain

Effective analgesia in neuropathic pain and other syndromes

Antidepressants are used widely to treat symptoms other than depression, many of which fit into a general category of pain. They include neuropathic pain (postherpetic neuralgia, diabetic neuropathy (p 827) (1)), irritable bowel syndrome, temporomandibular joint dysfunction, atypical facial pain, and fibromyalgia. In Britain no antidepressant is licensed for these indications. Do they work?

There is strong evidence from systematic reviews of randomised trials that tricyclic antidepressants are effective treatments for several of these conditions.(2) (3) (4) For established postherpetic neuralgia, tricyclic antidepressants seem to be the only drugs of proved benefit,4 and the number needed to treat to achieve at least 50% pain relief after three to six weeks compared with placebo was 2.3 (95% confidence interval 1.7 to 3.3).2 This means that two patients in five will achieve this (high) level of relief who would not have done so with placebo. Numbers needed to treat of two to three compare well with the most effective analgesics in acute pain, and with anticonvulsants in neuropathic pain.(5)

Figure 1 shows results from individual randomised trials of diabetic neuropathy and postherpetic neuralgia, each point representing one randomised trial.2 All the points fall in the upper segment, showing treatment to be better than placebo. Overall, about 50-90% of patients can expect to achieve at least 50% pain relief with antidepressants, while others will achieve a lower level of relief that may still be worth while for them.

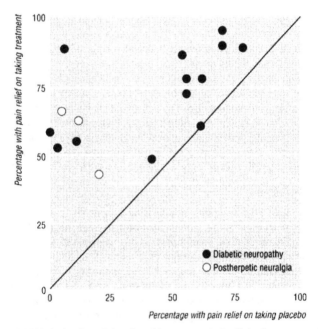

Figure 1: L'Abbé plot for trials of antidepressants in diabetic neuropathy and postherpetic neuralgia, showing percentage of patients achieving at least 50% pain relief when taking antidepressants versus placebo1

Antidepressants also work in other neuropathic pain syndromes. In 13 randomised studies of diabetic neuropathy the number needed to treat to achieve at least 50% pain relief was 3.0 (2.4 to 4), and in two studies of atypical facial pain it was 2.8 (2.0 to 4.7). The estimated number needed to treat from one study of pain after stroke was 1.7.3

The analgesic effects of antidepressants differ in several ways from classic descriptions of their action on depression itself. Amitriptyline, for example, has proved analgesic efficacy with a median preferred dose of 75 mg (with a clear dose response (6)) in a range of 25-150 mg daily. This range is lower than traditional doses for depression of 150-300 mg. The speed of onset of effect is much faster (one to seven days) than that reported in depression, and the analgesic effect is distinct from any effect on mood.(7)

The commonest adverse effects are drowsiness and dry mouth, which occur in one in three cases. About one in 30 patients has to stop taking the drug because of intolerable or unmanageable side effects. The profile of adverse effects is the same as when the drugs are used to treat depression.

Antidepressants have two roles in managing chronic pain. The primary role is when pain relief with conventional analgesics (from aspirin or paracetamol through to morphine) is inadequate or when pain relief is combined with intolerable or unmanageable adverse effects. The failure of conventional analgesics should justify a therapeutic trial of antidepressants, particularly if the pain is neuropathic (pain in a numb area). There used to be a dogma that the character of the neuropathic pain was predictive of response, so that burning pain should be treated with antidepressants and shooting pain with anticonvulsants. Max showed that this was wrong; in his study both burning and shooting pain responded to tricyclic antidepressants.(7)

A secondary role of antidepressants in treating chronic pain is their use in addition to conventional analgesics. This can be particularly effective in patients with cancer who have pain in multiple sites, some nociceptive and some neuropathic. Improved sleep is a huge bonus.

So which antidepressant should be chosen and at what dose? Tricyclic antidepressants have proved efficacy in chronic pain, but there is little evidence that one drug is better than another, though some patients troubled by adverse effects may benefit from changing drug. The common first choice is amitriptyline, with a starting dose of 25 mg (10 mg in frail patients) to be taken as a single night time dose one hour before lights out. We advise patients to increase the dose by 25 mg at weekly intervals until they either achieve pain relief or adverse effects become problematic. The maximum dose is 150 mg. Patients are warned to expect a dry mouth and drowsiness, which is why they should take the drug at night. If they are still drowsy first thing in the morning they should take the drug earlier in the evening.

There is no evidence that the newer antidepressants have greater analgesic effect than tricyclic drugs. The number needed to treat to achieve at least 50% pain relief was five for paroxetine and 15.3 for fluoxetine, while mianserin showed no difference from placebo.1 There is still insufficient evidence from trials to be sure about this. The lower incidence of adverse effects for selective serotonin reuptake inhibitors (fluoxetine and paroxetine) than with tricyclic drugs may make them worth trying for those patients who cannot take tricyclics because of adverse effects.

One obvious question is what happens in the long term. Most evidence of efficacy comes from short term trials (lasting weeks to months), and, although many patients continue to achieve pain relief with antidepressants for months to years, this is not true for everybody. Another puzzle is how antidepressants work as analgesics. The standard (but not compelling) explanation is that they act on descending tracts from the brain via noradrenaline and serotonin systems to modulate signalling of pain in the spinal cord. This sounds, and is, an unsatisfactory explanation. But in the meantime it is clear that antidepressants have an important role to play in relieving chronic pain.

Henry J McQuay, Clinical reader in pain relief, and R Andrew Moore, Consultant biochemist are at the Pain Research and Nuffield Department of Anaesthetics, University of Oxford, Oxford Radcliffe Hospital, The Churchill, Oxford OX3 7LJ

1. Milligan K. 'Prescribing antidepressants in general practice'. *BMJ*, 1997; 314:827-8.
2. McQuay HJ, Tramèr M, Nye BA, Carroll D, Wiffen PJ, Moore RA. 'A systematic review of antidepressants in neuropathic pain'. *Pain* 1996; 68:217-27.
3. Onghena P, Van Houdenhove B. 'Antidepressant-induced analgesia in chronic non-malignant pain: a meta-analysis of 39 placebo-controlled studies'. *Pain* 1992; 49:205-19.

4. Volmink J, Lancaster T, Gray S, Silagy C. 'Treatments of postherpetic neuralgia: A systematic review of randomized controlled trials'. *Fam Pract* 1996; 13:84-91.

5. McQuay H, Carroll D, Jadad AR, Wiffen P, 'Moore A. Anticonvulsant drugs for management of pain: a systematic review'. *BMJ,* 1995; 311:1047-52.

6. McQuay HJ, Carroll D, Glynn CJ. 'Dose-response for analgesic effect of amitriptyline in chronic pain'. *Anaesthesia* 1993; 48:281-5.

7. Max MB, Lynch SA, Muir J, Shoaf SF, Smoller B, Dubner R. 'Effects of desipramine, amitriptyline, and fluoxetine on pain in diabetic neuropathy'. *N Engl J Med* 1992; 326:1250-6.

Resource 7

How to hit pain before it hurts you

Painkillers a the time of your anaesthetic could be the best way to reduce the pain that seems inevitable after an operation – if the new findings about different types of pain are anything to go by

Twist your ankle and you feel a sharp, intense pain that grows worse in a matter of seconds and then nearly as rapidly begins to fade. In its place may come another sort of pain: a deeper, more diffuse, rather sickening pain that spreads steadily through the lower leg and foot. If you feel this second sort of pain, you know you are in trouble: you won't be able to walk normally for several days, perhaps a week.

The recognition that there is more than one basic kind of pain has led to a breakthrough in our ability to diagnose and treat a wide variety of pain symptoms. We now know that people experience different kinds of pain, caused by distinct mechanisms in the nervous system, and that each sort of pain demands its own unique form of relief.

The sharp, intense pain you feel as you first twist your ankle is an example of protective pain. This physiological sensation is a part of the body's normal sensitivity, on a par with perceptions of touch or warmth. This kind of pain is a vital early warning system, for we feel it specifically when nerve endings in our skin and internal organs detect something – be it mechanical, chemical or thermal – intense enough that it threatens to damage tissue.

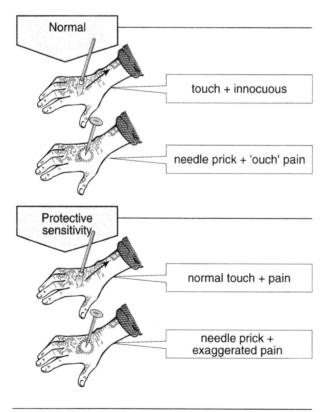

Figure 1: The pain that tries to protect: normally a light touch does not feel painful, but if the area has already been slightly injured, the body's protective mechanisms will make even a delicate paintbrush seem painful.

Such so-called "noxious' stimuli activate a set of highly specialised detectors located on the ends of special pain-generating sensory nerve cells, or neurons. These special sensory neurons, called nociceptors, translate noxious stimuli into electrical signals which then travel up the nerves to the spinal cord. There, they activate central sensory pathways which, in turn, send messages to particular regions of the brain. The end result is the conscious awareness of a sharp, clearly defined, well localised, unpleasant sensation.

Protective pain alerts the body to potential danger. It is accompanied by a reflex withdrawal of the part of the body in contact with the noxious stimulus, as well as more complicated responses such as cries, grimaces and perhaps even tears. We rapidly learn to predict what classes of stimuli are likely to produce this kind of pain response. Seeing a doctor approaching with a syringe and needle, touching a red hot metal bar or banging your head against a wooden beam – these all immediately lead you to anticipate the likely sensory outcome.

Protective pain, which I like to call the "ouch pain", was once thought to represent the beginning of a single continuous pain spectrum. But we now know that there is a second sort of pain, reparative pain, that is distinctly different. It is the dull, sickening, spreading sort of pain that sets in if you really have injured your ankle badly in that twist. Now it is too late for protection; the damage has been done. The acute trauma caused by falling awkwardly on your ankle has overwhelmed the body's protective mechanisms in that area.

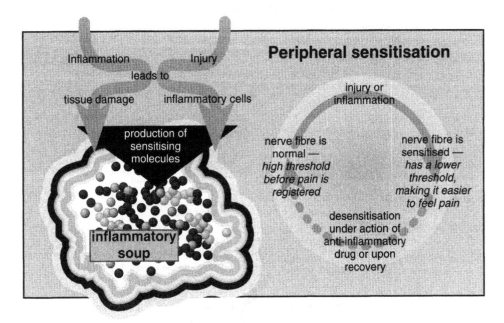

Figure 2: The pain which seeks to heal: the nerve fibres near the site of injury become more sensitive until the area is healed or by the pain is blocked by an anti-inflammatory drug.

The same thing can happen when an infection or an immune response sparks off a full-blown inflammation in a certain area, leading to tissue damage (see Figure 2). In both trauma and inflammation, the priority is to prevent further tissue damage and to promote healing and repair. The best solution is to avoid all stimuli and immobilise the whole organism, or at least the damaged body part, until the injury has healed. But how can we do this? Evolution has designed an ingenious mechanism, known as sensory hypersensitivity, which we experience as a kind of persistent pain while the problem area is healing. This can last several hours or several weeks, depending on the severity of the injury.

Neurons become extra sensitive

How is this achieved? Two mechanisms are at work. First, the nociceptors in the skin and internal organs become more sensitive, a process known as peripheral sensitisation. This causes the feeling of pain when bathing or showering after acute sun burn – what are usually pleasantly warm stimuli on the skin suddenly feel painful. Secondly, neurons in the spinal cord also become more sensitive than normal – the process of central sensitisation – and that means serious pain is in store.

Peripheral sensitisation generates hypersensitivity only in the immediate vicinity of any injured tissue, while central sensitisation causes a spread of extreme sensitivity, particularly to mechanical stimuli (try putting your weight on your bad ankle), far beyond the site of damage.

What is remarkable is that this tenderness is produced, not because of any change in the nociceptors, but because of changes in the sensitivity or excitability of neurons in the spinal cord. Even a gentle touch may now be painful. Thanks to the increased excitability of the spinal cord, innocuous inputs that would usually elicit only neutral or even pleasant sensations of touch or pressure now produce an abnormal feeling of pain.

Peripheral sensitisation is produced as a result of the local release of chemicals such as prostaglandins which effectively announce that tissue is damaged. Drugs that interfere with this prostaglandin production, and so reduce the inflammatory response – notably the non-steroidal anti-inflammatory-like drugs (NSAIDs) such as aspirin or ibuprofen – probably reduce pain because they block peripheral sensitisation.

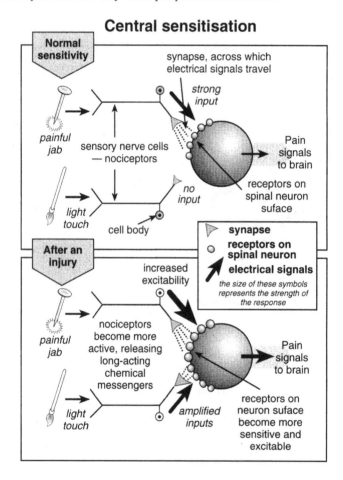

Figure 3: Overactive cells: nerve cells in the spinal cord can become sensitised by a biochemical cascade of long-acting neurotransmitters promoted by an over-active nociceptor near the injured site. The spinal neurons become even more excitable, and even light touches can seem painful.

Central sensitisation, on the other hand, is triggered in spinal neurons by the action of intensely active nociceptors (see Figure 3). These send signals down the nerve fibre to the terminal with the spinal neuron and long-acting chemical messengers are released across the synapse (the nerve to nerve junction). Studying these activities in my laboratory, and that of Anthony Dickenson at University College London, we have found that these messengers, known as neurotransmitters, in turn set off a complex biochemical cascade that, in the end, increases the excitability of the spinal neurons. Once this happens, inputs that the spinal neurons would normally ignore begin to elicit a vigorous response which, transmitted to the brain, results in a feeling of pain. The cellular processes involved are very like those involved in learning and memory; indeed, some scientists believe that pain hypersensitivity may represent the earliest form of neurons having any sort of memory.

Novel targets for new painkillers

Central sensitisation was first described in my laboratory in the early 1980s, and later in many laboratories in the USA, Germany, Sweden, Canada and here in the UK. This phenomenon has transformed approaches to managing inflammatory pain. For a start, it offers novel targets for the development of new painkillers that may work by reducing hypersensitivity in spinal neurons, and my colleagues and I and many drug companies are now searching for such analgesic agents. But even without new drugs, our greater understanding of the physiology of reparative pain already offers a new strategy for treating pain – the concept of pre-emptive analgesia (see also Box).

The idea is that much severe pain could be prevented from ever developing. If we could block the establishment of central sensitisation, we could stop extreme sensitivity before it kicks in. What is more, it should be easier to prevent this sort of pain than to try to treat it once it has become established.

Conventional therapy for acute pain consists of giving either aspirin-like NSAIDs – or morphine-like drugs to patients when they complain of pain. (Morphine and similar drugs act to prevent the release of the long-lasting neuro-transmitters which get the spinal neurons all fired up.) In pre-emptive analgesia, doctors give patients painkillers before the pain has a chance to set in. So a patient about to have abdominal surgery could be given morphine before or while they are anaesthetised.

Behind this novel approach lies the recognition that even under general anaesthesia, surgery can lead to central sensitisation: the sensory signals generated by cutting or cauterising tissue during surgery still excite the neurons in the spinal cord. We now know that during operations, spinal neurons become abnormally sensitive to all sensory signals, so that once patients come round from the anaesthesia, they feel pain even in response to normally innocuous inputs such a slight touch or pressure. Pre-emptive analgesia tries to prevent this from happening.

Clinical trials at University College Hospital, London in 1993 with Lesley Bromley showed that giving morphine to women before rather than during surgery reduced by about a third their need for painkillers after hysterectomies and also significantly reduced abdominal tenderness.

Other trials in Canada, the US and Denmark, which involved giving patients local anaesthetics to block sensory input from the wound site to the spinal cord, and morphine-like drugs also show promise. More trials are in progress to perfect this therapeutic strategy.

There is one final category of pain: the kind that follows damage to the nervous system itself, for instance nerve injury as after a car accident or bullet wound, or due to diseases such as diabetes. This generates a much more severe, potentially long-term pain, known as neuropathic pain. This final form of pain has nothing to do with protecting or repairing the body. It offers no biological advantage to the patient, and represents an abnormal response of the system when under extreme circumstances which then unfortunately persists. Like the pain associated with inflammation, neuropathic pain is caused by abnormal hypersensitivity of neurons in the spinal cord. Stimuli that would not normally produce pain begin to do so, and we no longer need noxious stimuli to evoke the sensation of pain.

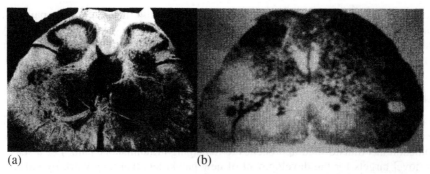

(a)   (b)

Figure 4: The connections that create pain: (a) shows a healthy spinal chord, with the normal nerve structure picked out. If damage to the nerves is particularly severe, not only will the spinal neurons become hypersensitive, but other nerves which normally sense feelings like touch and pressure, will rewire themselves to the pain-registering nerve fibres. The darker shapes picked out in (b) show where pain signals are being generated in the rewired region.

The terrible chronic pain associated with damage to the nervous system has two parts: a central component – structural and chemical changes within the central nervous system – and a peripheral component: changes in the damaged sensory neurons. But a key difference between the two is that nerve damage causes permanent changes in the way that peripheral sensory neurons are wired up, and so far, very little can be done to put things right (see Figure 4).

After peripheral nerve injury, for instance, the sensory fibres that normally signal the sensation of light touch grow away from their normal location in the spinal cord to a new site. Whether this happens relates to whatever fibres are damaged, and to the severity of the damage. There the fibres wrongly establish new connections with those neurons that normally receive inputs from nociceptors. This explains the exquisite sensitivity people with some forms of nerve damage have to the lightest of touches. This irreversible rewiring of the circuitry of this sensory pathway in the spinal cord appears to be responsible for the intractable nature of neuropathic pain and its resistance to all forms of conventional treatment. The rewiring is detectable a week after the initial nerve injury, and then remains for a long time. Indeed, we don't know whether this change is ever undone. Now we have defined the causes one of our goals is to attempt to prevent the establishment of these major structural changes. It would appear that we have a week within which to act.

The mainstays of pain management today remain aspirin-like NSAIDs and opiates such as morphine, both of whose medical credentials have emerged from experience in hospitals and not from scientific research. At last, however, thanks to our new-found understanding of the nature and mechanisms involved, we can begin to develop new treatments based on a rational appreciation of the processes lying at the root of severe and enduring pain.

Medical research and the assault on pain

About 10 per cent of the population suffer from chronic pain, pain that has lasted longer than several months. For perhaps four-fifths of these people, pain-relieving drugs will keep the problem under control, so that they can continue to lead their normal daily lives. But if the pain cannot be sorted out for the remainder, that adds up to 365 million days of pain per year. This degree of disability seriously affects these people's quality of life, as well as taking a huge economic toll in terms of lost employment and disability payments.

Twenty per cent of people with cancer have the worse kind of pain, neuropathic pain, (see Figure 4, main article), and this is extremely difficult to treat. There are also a huge number of patients in hospital for medical or surgical treatment whose pain control leaves much to be desired. A recent survey by Brian Jarman's team at St Mary's Hospital Medical School revealed that 33 per cent of those suffering pain were in pain all or most of the time, and 87 per cent of those with pain rated it as moderate to severe. Each year there are 3 million operations with general anaesthetics and, on average, each patient stays in hospital for three days. If pain relief after an operation could be improved, either as a result of the pre-emptive measures mentioned in the main article, or for other reasons, the cost of 9 million pain days to the National Health Service could be greatly reduced.

But how to tackle such a major medical problem? The first thing has to be to work across boundaries. Basic scientists in their laboratories need to collaborate with doctors and pain specialists in hospital, hospices, pain clinics and general practice. Over the last few years, dialogue between these groups has led to many new ideas. Researchers have identified a large number of targets for drug development, and our knowledge of how pain is transmitted and the possibilities for control has expanded greatly.

One problem, however, is the long time it takes for a new analgesic to be developed, trialled and then made available. Therefore our group, and a number of others around the country, are looking at drugs which are already licensed for other, non-pain-related reasons, to see whether they could have a role to play. Not only could these drugs be used on their own, but it should be possible to use studies on animals to predict which would work best in combinations, with reduced side effects. These could then be used as a basis for trials on humans.

A major challenge is to find ways of reducing central hypersensitivity (see Figure 3, main article), particularly when it has already set in. Drugs which could be valuable include those which block key pain receptors in hypersensitivity such as low doses of ketamine, normally used to in high doses as an anaesthetic and dextromethorphan, used as a cough suppressant. Many people who have had a limb amputated, perhaps after an accident, still have strong bursts of pain seemingly where the limb used to be. Reports suggest that low doses of ketamine stopped the phantom limb pains, and more work is now going on to see how this initial finding can be put to best use.

We now have an idea why certain types of pain do not respond well to opioid-type drugs, and we should be able to remedy this by combining morphine with a number of other drugs.

As well as treating established pain, if the transition from acute, treatable pain to pain which cannot be treated could be prevented, the benefits would be considerable. The increased costs in the hospital would be easily offset by long term benefits, both to the patients and their families, and to the national economy.

We continue to need a concerted effort across all disciplinary boundaries. Here at the Thomas Lewis Pain Research Centre we work closely with the Anaesthetics Department at University College Hospital, London. Maria Fitzgerald and I have colleagues at Great Ormond Street Hospital collaborating on the particular problem of pain control in infants and children.

A key role for health professionals will be to quantify the problem. What are the problems? How big are they, and how well are they tackled at present. The Pain Relief Unit in Oxford is working on answers to these questions which will guide the direction of pain research in the future.

Anthony Dickenson

Clifford Woolf is a Professor of Neurobiology in the Department of Anatomy and Developmental Biology at University College London. He runs a multidisciplinary research group using molecular biological, neurochemical, electrophysiological, neuroanatomical and behavioural techniques to study pain mechanisms, as well as collaborating with clinical colleagues in running clinical pain trials. He is a director of the newly established Thomas Lewis Pain Research Centre at University College London, which aims to establish an active partnership between basic scientists, clinicians and the pharmaceutical industry to devise new and more effective approaches for managing pain.

Professor Anthony Dickenson, based at the Department of Pharmacology at University College London, is co-director of the Thomas Lewis Pain Research Centre. His interests are in the pharmacology of pain transmission and its control.

Further reading

Richmond, C.E., Bromley, L.M., Woolf, C.J. (1994) 'Preoperative morphine pre-empts postoperative pain', *Lancet* 342; 73-75.

Wall, P.D., Melzack, R. (1994), *Textbook of Pain*, 3rd edn, Churchill Livingstone.

Woolf, C.J. (1983) 'Evidence for a central component of post-injury pain hypersensitivity', *Nature* 306: 688-688.

Woolf, C.J., Shortland, P., Coggeshall, R.E. (1992) 'Peripheral nerve injury triggers central sprouting of myelinated afferents', *Nature* 355: 75-77.